Awareness and Influence in Health and Social Care

HOW YOU CAN REALLY MAKE A DIFFERENCE

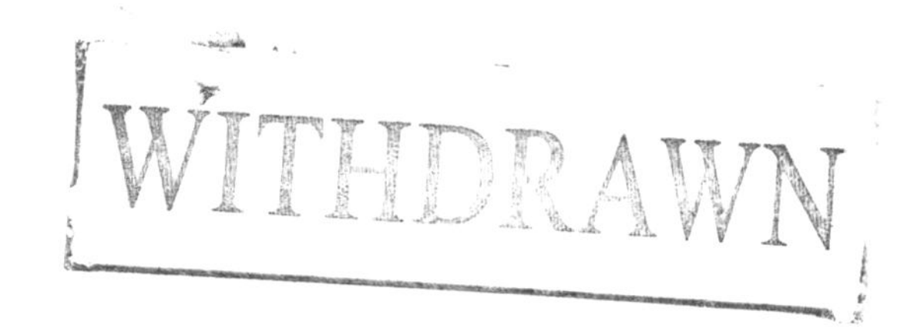

ROSEMARY COOK

Director
The Queen's Nursing Institute

Radcliffe Publishing
Oxford • Seattle

Radcliffe Publishing Ltd
18 Marcham Road
Abingdon
Oxon OX14 1AA
United Kingdom

www.radcliffe-oxford.com
Electronic catalogue and worldwide online ordering facility.

British Library Cataloguing in Publication Data

A catalogue record for this book is available from the British Library.

ISBN-10 1 84619 075 4
ISBN-13 978 1 84619 075 9

Typeset by Egan Reid Ltd, Auckland, New Zealand
Printed and bound by TJ International Ltd, Padstow, Cornwall

For Alison,
my original role model,
mentor and more.

Contents

About the author

Rosemary Cook is the Director of The Queen's Nursing Institute. Her professional experience includes clinical work in primary care as a practice nurse, and management and facilitation roles in health authorities. She worked at the Department of Health for five years on a range of nursing and primary care-related policies.

Rosemary is the author of two other books, and is a prolific writer and columnist for nursing, management and GP journals. She is a regular conference speaker and workshop leader. Rosemary has two grown-up daughters and lives in Cheshire with her partner.

Acknowledgements

I would like to thank all the friends, colleagues and new contacts who provided the helpful hints on awareness and influence that appear throughout this book. As well as enriching and enlivening the text, they have enabled me to expand my networks, particularly with new contacts amongst healthcare scientists, allied health professionals and social care colleagues.

I would also like to thank the following people who have given permission for their quotations to be used throughout this book:

- Sue Boran, Senior Lecturer, London South Bank University/Secretary, Association of District Nurse Educators
- Kay East, Head of Allied Health Professions, Department of Health, England
- Judith Ellis, Director of Nursing and Human Resources, Great Ormond Street Hospital for Children NHS Trust
- Jayne Elton, Specialist Practitioner and Lead Practice Nurse, Frome
- Monica Fletcher, Chief Executive, Education for Health (formerly National Respiratory Training Centre)
- Jean Gray, Editor, *Nursing Standard*
- Judy Hargadon, Chief Executive, School Food Trust
- Suzanne Hilton, Commissioning and Performance Manager, Allied Health Professionals
- Deb Lapthorne, Director of Public Health, Plymouth Teaching Primary Care Trust/Plymouth City Council
- Alexandra Lejeune, Senior Occupational Therapist, South East London
- Rosalynde Lowe, Chair, The Queen's Nursing Institute
- Helen McCloughry, Head of Rehabilitation and Intermediate Care, Nottingham City Primary Care Trust
- Sandra Mellors, Head of Physiotherapy Service, Tower Hamlets Primary Care Trust
- Helen Mould, Head of Adult Speech and Language Therapy, Birmingham/Chair SHA AHPs and Health Care Scientists' network
- Alison Norman, Director of Nursing and Operations, The Christie Hospital NHS Trust
- Sue Norman, Trustee, The Burdett Trust for Nursing

- Joanna Parker, Head of Safer Practice, National Patient Safety Agency
- Anne Pearson, Practice Development Manager, The Queen's Nursing Institute
- Liz Plastow, UK Nursing and Midwifery Council
- Julia Quickfall, Nurse Director, The Queen's Nursing Institute, Scotland
- Christine Singleton, Clinical Specialist (FES) & West Midlands Regional Spasticity Project Manager
- Penny Spreadbury, Head of Service, Nottingham Back Team
- Barbara Stuttle, Director of Primary Care and Modernisation, Thurrock Primary Care Trust
- Judith Whittam, Health and Social Care Change Agent Team, Department of Health, Engand
- Maureen Williams, Head of Primary and Social Care, London South Bank University
- Fran Woodard, Director, Modernisation Initiative, Guy's and St Thomas' NHS Trust

Introduction

This is a book about the skills, habits and behaviours that make people influential. Why you want to be influential doesn't matter. You may be really keen to improve care locally, earn fifty thousand a year or finish your career as a 'sir' or a 'dame'. It makes no difference to the key skills you need to acquire.

The good news is that influence is not just for 'senior' people, or people in specific jobs, any more. The old hierarchies are breaking down, 'frontline' expertise is valued by policy makers more than ever before, and London is no longer the centre of the universe for influence on health and social care policy and practice. You can be well-known and influential from anywhere, including home, and neither working part-time, taking career breaks, nor restricted mobility is a barrier to this.

The other good news is that anyone can do it – if they are prepared to put some personal effort into it. People sometimes ask how they can acquire 'strategic thinking' or 'strategic awareness' as if it is an all-or-nothing entity. In fact, it is more like an edifice built from smaller blocks of information, skills and opportunities. Together, they combine to create strategic thinking and awareness – as shown in the figure below. Information can be acquired. Skills can be learned. Opportunities can be created. This means that it is possible for everyone to become strategic thinkers, and exert influence where it is needed. The aim of this book is to help you to acquire, learn and create, in order to influence.

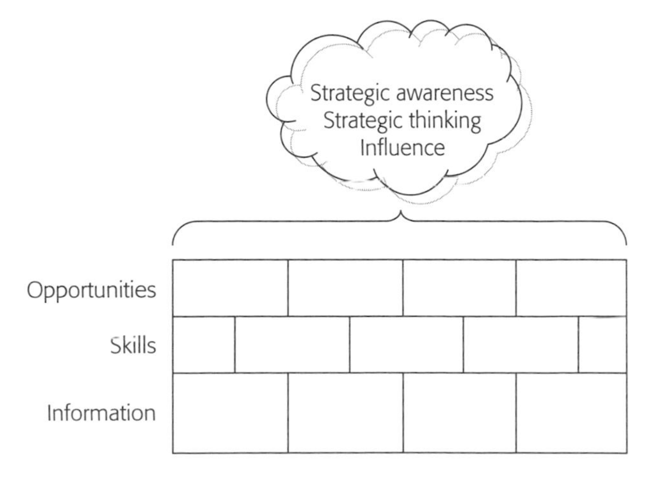

This book does not tell you the right way, the only way or even the best way to go about gaining influence, and its essential precursor, awareness. But it does contain some tried and tested tips, from a wide range of influential people, as well as my own experience. These should help you to adopt approaches that are likely to be successful – rather than those that automatically close doors.

Five simple guidelines summarise the advice in this book. You need to:

- do the simple things well
- invest your own time
- treat everything as an opportunity
- treat other people well
- understand the context as well as the issues.

And if you don't read any further, your action plan should be to:

- brush up your IT skills
- write some articles
- expand your network
- get a mentor
- join or form a group.

If you do read on, and take time to look at the personal development exercises and checklists for action, I believe you will find it remarkably easy to build your awareness, and to influence those policies and practices that will really make a difference.

SECTION 1

Principles

CHAPTER 1

How to use this book: scope and approach

This is a book about increasing your awareness and your influence. It has three key aims:

- to help you to find new ways to expand your knowledge of practice, policy and the service in which you work
- to suggest how you can build expertise in some key practical skills needed for influence
- to show how you can use these skills to increase your influence on the people who develop health policy, practice and the health service.

Since everyone starts with a different combination of experience, personality and ambition, it would be impossible for the contents of this book to be exactly right for every person using it. Parts of it will seem obvious and unnecessary to some people, while for others, the same ideas and suggestions will be exciting and challenging. What is already everyday behaviour to one person is a leap in the dark for another. There is no 'one size fits all' solution for success.

So one way to use this book would be to look down the list of contents, and dip into those sections that seem to have something new to offer you. Alternatively, it can be read from beginning to end, as consolidation of your existing skills and practices, but with the expectation of finding at least one or two new ideas for further professional development.

Throughout the book you will find devices to help you relate the contents of each section to your own situation. These include:

- '*mirror moments*': for reflection on the issue under discussion, its impact on you and your practice, and your attitude to it
- *personal development exercises*: tasks aimed specifically at exercising a particular skill
- '*portfolio pointers*': ideas for recording your actions in your personal professional portfolio
- *checklists for action*: things you could do to increase your awareness, develop your networks and enhance your influence, even before you finish the book.

These devices are all aimed at making the book a useful tool for development, rather than simply an interesting read. Try to find time to stop and undertake the activities suggested – they will make sure that you finish the book already more aware, and more influential, than you started, and with an improved professional portfolio to prove it.

- The '*need to know*' boxes provide additional information on relevant topics. If you have ever wondered what 'Chatham House Rules' means, where to get support for 'whistleblowing' or which topics are exempt from disclosure under the Freedom of Information Act, this is where you will find the information.

Throughout the book are quotes from key individuals who are already policy makers, influencers, professional leaders and role models across the health and social care spectrum. Their advice on the topics covered in this book adds weight and substance to the topics discussed.

Together, the different tools and devices in this book should provide you with both the recipe and the ingredients for a more aware and influential future.

What is covered in the book?

There is an almost endless list of topics that could be useful to health and social care workers looking for help to develop skills and enhance their development. This book covers many of the more common questions that are asked on leadership courses and in individual meetings with professionals who are keen to develop their influence, but are not sure how to proceed. These include:

- how do I build up a professional network?
- how do I spread good practice outside of my unit?
- how do I record 'influence' in my personal professional profile?
- how should I contribute to a strategy meeting, a meeting with a government minister, or a professional conference?
- could I write an article for a professional journal?
- who is 'in charge' of policy on my particular topic?
- is it possible to combine an influential career with a family?
- can I have influence without leaving the workplace?
- what if my employer is not supportive?
- what will happen if I speak out?

These topics form the backbone of subsequent sections, together with other tips and topics that contribute to the development of awareness and influence.

Who is it for?

It will be clear from these sample questions that the advice given – and other topics and skills discussed in this book – are applicable across the whole spectrum of the health and social care professions. I have used examples of nurses, midwives, allied health professionals, healthcare scientists and social care workers randomly through the text: wherever one group is mentioned, the text is usually applicable to other workers in the health and social care system too.

It will also apply to professionals of different grades, positions and practice areas, working for different employers. As the introduction made clear, the need for a book like this arises partly because traditional hierarchies are being removed or inverted, role models are harder to find, and the potential for national exposure and influence, regardless of 'status', has never been greater. So there is no particular level of professional at which this book is aimed: it is equally relevant to the student and the director, the practitioner and the service commissioner.

Where does this advice come from?

The source of the advice, ideas and tips in this book is much broader than my own experience. I have brought together what I have learned from many other influential people whom I have watched and emulated over the years: midwives, managers, doctors, nurses, civil servants and scientists. It is their amalgamated wisdom, leadership, example and support that have been summarised here, together with my own experiences and mistakes, to produce a toolkit for you to use and to pass on.

It is important to stress that the ideas in this book do not necessarily represent the best or only way to go about expanding your awareness and influence. There are many other ways to achieve the same ends, and you may have found your own equally valid and successful approach. But these ideas have all worked for someone, in some circumstances, so they are worthy of inclusion on their own merits.

The approach

This book does not contain any theory. It does not explain models of leadership, or the empirical basis of networking. It is practical, and practice based, in the widest sense: real world practice, in all fields, not only clinical practice. If it sometimes appears didactic – 'do this, do that' – then this is just shorthand for 'you could consider . . .' or 'why not try . . .?' View all suggestions through the window of your own situation, ambition, experience and talents, weigh up the advice, and choose those elements of it that you want to try. Above all, if you want to increase your awareness and influence, make a start – do something!

PORTFOLIO POINTER

Reading this book, undertaking some of the development activities contained in it and applying them to your own practice or area of work, could be recorded in your personal professional portfolio as a contribution to meeting your continuing professional development (CPD) requirements. There are many specific suggestions for what to record in your portfolio in the course of the following chapters. If you don't have a portfolio, this would be a good time to start one!

Some professional organisations sell them, or give them to members. Otherwise an ordinary ring binder file will do as a convenient place to keep together your important professional information. *See* Box 1.1 for what sort of documents and records to keep in your portfolio.

BOX 1.1 What to put in a personal professional file (portfolio)

A personal portfolio will usually contain:

- qualification certificates
- evidence of other training courses or events attended
- reflections on learning or further training needs
- reflections on future career or job aspirations, and plans to achieve them.

It could contain:

- copies of your latest CV
- programmes of conferences you have attended/spoken at
- articles or letters you have had published
- thank you letters from groups or committees you contributed to
- appraisals from your current job
- contact network maps.

CHAPTER 2

Awareness and influence: what do they mean?

Awareness in health and social care comes in two forms:

- awareness of knowledge for practice, and
- awareness of the context of practice.

Knowledge for practice – the facts, figures, theories, judgements and ideas used every day in the care of patients or clients, or the education, management and development of practice and practitioners – is not the focus of this book. That is the kind of knowledge gained in formal education, through courses and reflection on practice, or through reading journals or textbooks. But it can be knowledge gained and used in isolation, focused sharply on the daily task. It is essential for practice, but it will not necessarily take the practitioner outside of their practice to influence others.

Awareness of the context of practice is different. Knowing the context is like looking up from the wound dressing to take in the whole patient. It is seeing the daily task – clinical or otherwise – as part of a bigger picture. It is a kind of professional holism, rather than a 'job-focused' approach. And, for reasons that will be discussed more in the next section, it is an essential prerequisite for influence.

MIRROR MOMENT

Stop and reflect on this. Do you concentrate solely on your knowledge for practice, reading clinical or technical articles but skipping over news and analysis sections of journals? Are you proud of the fact that you just get on with the job, and don't bother with the journals at all? Or do you like to hear about how other people act in similar roles to yours, and to know what is happening in other parts of your organisation? Be honest with yourself: what is your response to the idea of expanding your awareness beyond the boundaries of your daily work?

Kinds of awareness

Awareness can be divided into any number of arbitrary categories – the possibilities are endless! But for simplicity, think of awareness in four domains: professional awareness, clinical awareness, organisational awareness and policy awareness. These domains, and some of the contextual issues in each category, are shown in Box 2.1.

BOX 2.1 Domains of awareness

Professional

- Who sets the standards for practice and conduct for your professional or occupational group?
- How many members of your group work in the NHS and how many in independent health and social care?
- What is your union/professional association most concerned about at present?

Clinical

- Who are the leading people in your field?
- Where is innovative/leading edge practice happening?
- What is the next 'breakthrough' technology likely to be?
- How many people locally and nationally are in the client group you deal with?

Organisational

- Who heads up your service in your organisation?
- Which board member has responsibility for it?
- How much money does the organisation spend on your area of practice?

Policy

- Which government department makes the policy decisions that most affect your area of work?
- What is the policy issue of the moment?
- What impact will it have if it is implemented locally?

PERSONAL DEVELOPMENT EXERCISE

Look at Box 2.1 and consider which domain you currently have most awareness in, and in which you are least aware. Take the one you are most interested in, and think about one or two of the context issues: could you confidently give this sort of information to a colleague, if asked? Then choose one of the areas in which you are least aware, and commit yourself to finding out something new in this area within the week.

Active awareness

Awareness may be about knowing, but it is not solely a passive, cerebral thing. You need to be active to be aware: reading widely, talking to people, listening, making phone calls, taking notes – and many other activities. There is more about this in Section 2, and these actions can lead to more actions, aimed at acquiring new skills or 'knowledge for practice', as a result of your awareness. For example, if your clinical awareness tells you that genetic causes of illness and susceptibility to illness are becoming increasingly well-recognised, and patients are asking about them, you might decide that you need to refresh your knowledge of genetic inheritance. Or your actions might be aimed at increasing your influence. If your policy awareness identifies the expanding role of healthcare workers in prescribing, you might dust off your dissertation on the topic, update it, and look for an appropriate person to talk to in order to influence that policy development. The relationship between awareness and influence will be explored more in the next chapter (*see* p. 11).

Here is a real example: a health visitor approached me on an exhibition stand at a national conference, and said that she was interested in working for the Department of Health on a secondment. This was an excellent example of opportunistic networking. We talked about working for the Department, and she was rather dismayed to learn about the degree to which Department officials use email for internal communications and the development of written documents. She had little access to computers, and was not used to working in this way. So my suggestion was that she should set out to obtain this skill while waiting for a secondment opportunity to arise. Her awareness of her development needs, and her action to meet them, will make her much more likely to get that secondment position and be able to influence health policy.

PERSONAL DEVELOPMENT EXERCISE

Look again at Box 2.1 and this time list the domains of awareness in the order of their importance *to you*. This will depend on your hopes and ambitions, and will help you decide where you will focus your efforts in subsequent personal development exercises. Now jot down your personal ambitions for the next year, and the longer term.

Ambitions

Bear in mind that your hopes and ambitions may be internally or externally focused. An internal focus is on you. You may want:

- a higher status job, or a position in a national organisation
- to be regarded as an expert in your field by your peers, or seen as the 'best' or most senior person by your patients, or to have more letters after your name
- to be sought out, to have your work or opinions valued
- more money, benefits, travel or autonomy
- a chance to change direction in your career
- a network of well-known contacts
- to be invited to award ceremonies and gala dinners.

Or, your ambitions may be externally focused. You may want to:

- improve the experience of your patients, or help your unit provide even better care
- help more other professionals to qualify, or develop, or succeed in other ways
- add something to the development of your profession
- make the health and care system better, more efficient, or more patient focused
- draw attention to problems or deficiencies in care, to protect people
- share good practice from your area of work.

In reality, of course, most people have a mixture of both internal and external ambitions – though few people are very honest about this. At one extreme, there are people who claim that they want nothing for themselves, they just want to make things better for their patients. They manage to imply that they would happily work for nothing, but rarely do. At the other extreme are the people who openly say they intend to get to 'the top', whatever that means to them, as fast as possible. You can almost hear their professional engine running from the day they enter training, and people who worked with them in their early years still have the footprints on their shoulders. Most people fall somewhere in the middle of this continuum, combining genuinely altruistic hopes for their profession and their patients with a healthy amount of ambition for themselves. Section 2 will explore further the link between awareness and the achievement of ambitions.

Influence

Influence is about helping to bring about changes, to policies, actions, attitudes or behaviours, *through mechanisms other than direct action*. If you throw a bedpan against the wall in frustration, you are not influencing it to achieve that trajectory, you are just plain chucking it! Similarly if you are in charge of a unit and you rule that staff will work self-rostered flexible hours, that is not influence. But if you attend a trust meeting on implementing the 'Improving Working Lives' strategy, and you present data, information and arguments that convince some sceptical managers of the benefits to the organisation of allowing flexible working, that is influence. 'Might' may be 'right', but influence is more impressive.

The great thing about influence is that it is not tied to position, status or profile. You can be influential in any post, any time, anywhere. It is up to you to decide how far you want to develop your influence, and in which direction. The domains of influence are the same as those for awareness: that is, they are innumerable, but can be categorised in many different ways for convenience.

If you want to influence clinical practice, or education or research, you can. If you want to influence health policy, or the workings of the NHS, you can. As the introduction made clear, there has never been a time when frontline health workers were offered more influence in all these, and many more, areas. So, the opportunities are there – this book aims to provide the tools for the job of developing awareness and influence, to take full advantage of these opportunities.

CHAPTER 3

Awareness and influence: the vital link

The point of linking awareness with influence is so that *you know what you are talking about when you try to influence people.* If you respond to a Department of Health consultation document on, for example, changes in professional regulation, or a new strategy for the care of vulnerable adults, and your response demonstrates your ignorance of the current situation, then your views on the future are unlikely to be taken seriously. Awareness and influence are inextricably linked. If you want to be able to change things where you work, or question the way the health service works, or influence the way services are provided to a particular group of vulnerable people, then you have to start from a position of awareness.

MIRROR MOMENT

Think about times when you have spoken out to try to influence an individual, or a meeting. Can you think of a time when you were 'put down' by someone pointing out that action was already underway, or the issue had already been raised, or another development would make your idea redundant? Avoiding these embarrassing moments is what awareness is all about.

Avoiding exposure

Most of us have experienced this at some time. It is embarrassing and demotivating, and makes it very tempting to adopt a 'lying low' strategy, and leave any attempt to change or influence to other people. But the key to avoiding being exposed to a 'put down' in such situations is developing your awareness. If you know what is happening in other parts of the organisation, in other organisations or services, or nationally, then you are far less likely to find yourself in such a position.

This doesn't mean you have to know everything about everything before you open your mouth. With experience (and the techniques and tips described in this book) you will very quickly know the shortcuts to such awareness. You will have:

- the habit of reading appropriate background
- the knowledge of where key facts can be found

- a network of good contacts to check out views with, and get different perspectives from
- techniques for storing and building on this information
- an organised approach to finding and using opportunities to influence, so that you use your awareness to greatest effect.

Using the awareness tool

Awareness is a tool, not an end in itself – but many people do not bother to acquire the awareness they need. It is astonishing how many people go into situations poorly prepared and ill-informed when they are seeking to influence other people and events. Even a small amount of preparation can greatly increase your awareness, and make you look very good in contrast to these people. If you put reasonable effort into raising your awareness of relevant issues, you will be not one or two, but probably ten steps ahead of others.

Having some awareness of the background to an issue does not of course mean that you are better able to make government policy on it than anyone else. But it does mean that you can try to influence, alongside other people who also have their pieces of the awareness jigsaw, and so affect the final picture.

The key is how you use the awareness tool. Just as you would not set out to adjust the solar panel on a space station with a screwdriver from B&Q, so you need to be aware of the limits and uses of your awareness of a topic. Trying to influence without

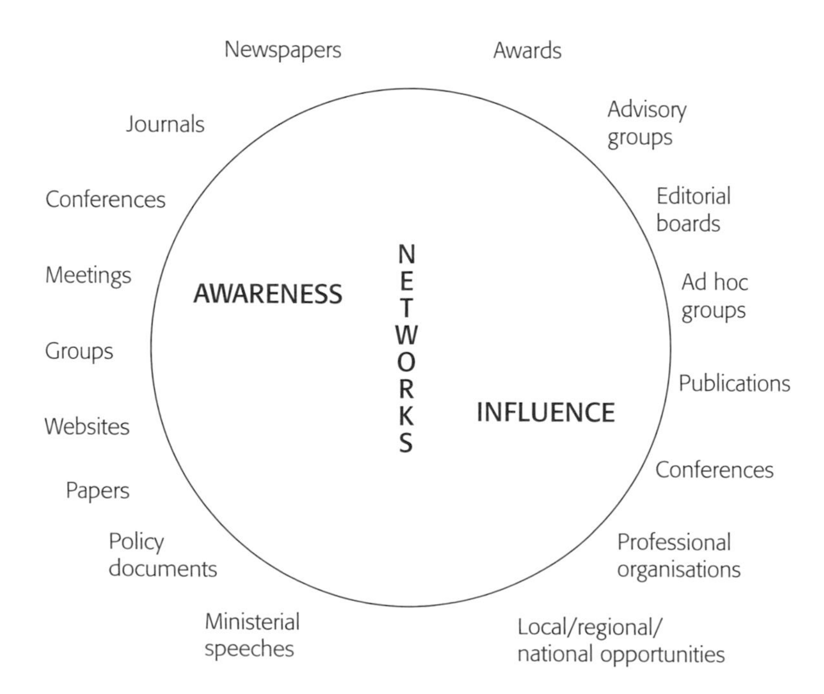

Figure 3.1 Awareness, influence and networks

any awareness would be like trying to finish the International Space Station with your bare hands!

One other vital distinction: awareness is not the same as opinion. You may have a detailed and cogent series of opinions about genetic engineering, but these will not be influential if you have no actual awareness of the subject, and the ethical, technological and professional issues surrounding it. In newspaper terms, it is the difference between a ranting tabloid column that has a transient interest for readers who share the same opinions, and a reasoned argument in a better quality paper that is noted by policy makers.

In practical terms, the link between awareness and influence is often in your networks. Having acquired a greater awareness of the topic through the people that you network with, it is usually other people in your network who give you the opportunity to use that tool to influence events. This connection is illustrated in Figure 3.1.

CHAPTER 4

Motivation to develop awareness and influence

MIRROR MOMENT

What is it that makes you interested in this book? What do you want as a reward for the effort you are putting in? Brainstorm the list first: is it a new job that you want? Appreciation within your own organisation? An award? Higher status? More money? A well-known name? Then rank the factors on your list in order of importance to you. This will help you to choose the most appropriate and effective activities and approaches later.

Understanding your motivation

Knowing your own motivation, and what you want to achieve, is particularly important because the first rule of influence is that you have to invest up front. No-one will pay you to read in your spare time, or be impressed by all the background knowledge and awareness you have that you don't have an opportunity to spell out in detail at a meeting. Unless there is something in this for you, something that you alone can identify and enjoy, you will find it hard to keep up the investment required. Remember, awareness is only a tool: unless you are very clear about the furniture you intend to build with it, shopping for a drill can be a very tedious and soul-destroying business.

CHAPTER 5

Dimensions of awareness and influence: your choice

It is vital to believe that you can be as influential as you choose to be – and you are free to choose a lot or a little. There is nothing wrong with saying 'I just want to change things in the organisation I work for' or 'I'm prepared to put this much of my time and effort into changing things in my bit of the health service, but the rest of my energy is for my family/hobby/model railway collection'. Equally, there is nothing wrong with saying 'I intend to be a well-known name in critical care nursing' or 'I want to be the keynote speaker at a professional conference/Chief Healthcare Scientist for Scotland/the youngest professor of social care in the UK'. That is your choice.

But it would be wrong to say 'I can't influence anything until my children are grown up', or 'My organisation is so hierarchical, there is no way I'll be in a position of influence for another decade'. Both technology and the radical redesign of health service careers now provide much greater opportunities for anyone who wants to take them. The key is what you choose to take from those tools and opportunities on offer.

MIRROR MOMENT

Think about your present job, whether in the home or in an organisation, in terms of your influence. How do you feel about your current level of influence? Who or what do you consider is responsible for your current situation? Looking at the domains of awareness described in Box 2.1 (*see* p. 8), in which domain are you going to choose to have influence?

CHAPTER 6

Key principles and steps to success

Principles

Here are seven key principles that apply to the business of building your awareness and increasing your influence:

To *build your awareness*, you need to:

- be prepared to invest your own time, energy and goodwill to succeed
- use all your resources: spare time, 'down time', curiosity, cunning, and cheek
- always know your ground before you act (awareness before influence).

To *increase your influence*, you need to:

- check out and obey the ground rules – about confidentiality, reliability, deadlines etc
- consciously plan to give more than you take
- recognise that influence is organic – it grows with care, and withers without it
- be 'bloody, bold and resolute' (as Shakespeare put it in *Macbeth*) – persistence and resilience are important
- grow a thick skin – you will need it.

Let's look at these more closely. First, investing in your awareness. There is no question that making yourself more aware takes up more time and energy than simply being a passive recipient of information. You have to make time to read, you have to bother to ask someone for an explanation, you have to make the effort to print off a policy paper from a website. And you may do all these things for months before you feel that you have a real opportunity to influence. But if you don't put anything in, you will not get anything out. And there is no predictable, direct relationship between what you put in and what you get out. The opportunities you do get may well be unexpected, and apparently unrelated to your investment. But what you have learned, practised, experienced or discovered about yourself while investing in your awareness will affect the way you respond to those opportunities.

Using all your resources to build your awareness is a way of getting maximum value from this investment. You don't have to set aside four hours a fortnight for 'awareness building' (though if you can, do it!). Instead, use a few minutes' spare time here and there; for example:

- if a meeting is late starting, use those few minutes to talk to someone you don't know, and find out something about their job or their views
- use a train journey, dentist's waiting room or wet Saturday afternoon to read an article, think through an issue or note down a contact number.

Time is not the only resource you can use. Exercise your curiosity: rather than simply wonder what an unknown financial term means, look it up or ask. Rather than let a casual reference go by, ask for the full details so you can look it up. Use all the facilities available to you to legitimately save your own time and effort. Libraries are often a greatly underused resource, with highly skilled people who can teach new IT skills, perform literature searches, track down references and photocopy articles. Similarly, experts in all fields are usually genuinely keen to share their knowledge. Trust audit departments, clinical governance leads, and technicians of all sorts are often extremely helpful. Seeing every job and every task within it as an opportunity to learn and expand your awareness quickly becomes a habit, and soon makes the whole business less of a conscious effort.

Knowing your ground is about having an appropriate degree of awareness before you act. It is the difference between dashing off a letter to a health minister to say 'Nurses in the community ought to be able to sign death certificates' and knowing the reasons why this does not happen, which other government departments are involved in the issue, and why there might be concern about a relaxation in the rules on death certification. Acting without awareness damages the credibility of not only the individual concerned, but the profession they represent as well.

BOX 6.1 Need to know: The Chatham House Rule

You may hear the expression 'Chatham House rules' used at a meeting. This phrase originated in 1927 with the Royal Institute of International Affairs, based in Chatham House in London. The Institute is a membership organisation that analyses international issues. The Rule (there is only one) was refined in 1997 and 2002. It states that: 'When a meeting, or part thereof, is held under the Chatham House Rule, participants are free to use the information received, but neither the identity nor the affiliation of the speaker(s), nor that of any other participant, may be revealed'. Its aim is to encourage openness and sharing of information by allowing anonymity to the speakers. It also allows people to give their own views as opposed to those of their organisation. *See* www.chathamhouse.org.uk/index.php?id=14.

Using the Chatham House Rule is of course different from saying that nothing said or heard in the meeting can be repeated outside; if this degree of confidentiality is required, it must be respected absolutely. If in doubt, check with the chair.

When you are trying to influence events or people, knowing and obeying the ground rules is vital. Sometimes these will be very clear: the requirements of confidentiality

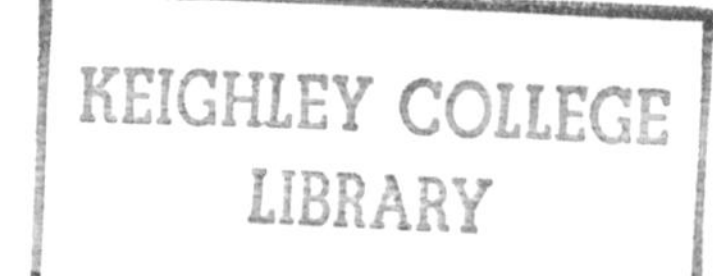

are often explicitly stated, either in writing on a document or verbally at a meeting. Be sure you understand what they mean, and if you are not sure, ask specifically at the start of the meeting (*see* Box 6.1).

Obeying the rules of confidentiality is absolutely essential. Whether it is a 'leak' from a policy meeting with Department of Health officials, from a trust meeting or a clinical supervision session, which may have political, financial, industrial relations or professional consequences, organisations take such breaches very seriously. Apart from any sanction that may be applied to you in the individual circumstances, you are unlikely ever to be invited to participate again if you are considered untrustworthy.

Reliability applies to more than just confidentiality. It is about being reliable in doing what you say you will do, whether it is passing on a contact name, setting up a meeting, or canvassing others' views. As a basic code of conduct:

- if you are not sure you can do something, don't say that you will
- don't be pressured into promising what you may not be able to deliver
- if you genuinely can't deliver something you have agreed to, contact the individual or chair of the group concerned as soon as possible, and explain – don't just hope they'll forget
- treat even relatively small tasks seriously – they are important to the person who asked you to do them
- give these 'extracurricular' tasks a fair position in your list of priorities – don't put them to the bottom of your in-tray when you return to work and say 'my proper job must come first'. Remember – if you can't give them the attention they deserve, don't take them on in the first place.

Too often people proclaim themselves to be keen to get involved, then fail to turn up at meetings, don't read the papers, or return work long after a deadline. They damage their own credibility, and their profession's.

This is a version of the other deadly sin to avoid: failing to balance give and take. If you take the kudos of being on a national advisory group, you must give the work, time and effort that the group requires. If you take information or advice from people in your network, you must give them, or other contacts, the benefit of your experience and knowledge when they ask. This is not only fair and right: it is itself an investment in your network, and so a way of continuing to build and nurture your own awareness and influence.

Being 'bloody, bold and resolute' is sometimes necessary. Influence rarely comes uninvited, which means that you have to put yourself forward, ask, offer, and risk being rebuffed. It does not mean barging and bullying your way to the forefront – this would demonstrate a lack of awareness of appropriate behaviour and skills that would almost guarantee closed doors. But it can be difficult even to push politely if you are naturally shy, you are limited by other circumstances, or if you feel unsupported by key people in your life or work. The techniques and tips in this book should demonstrate that none of these obstacles are insuperable.

The thick skin requirement is the other side of the 'boldness' coin. There is no doubt that putting your head above the parapet, to express an opinion, argue a case, push for a change or stand up for a principle, can be uncomfortable. There are always people who will criticise you, dislike you and even try to discredit you for doing so. The more influence you have, the more strongly some people will dislike you, and what you are doing. Some of these people will be close to you, personally or professionally. Others will be total strangers, or professional acquaintances, whose strength of feeling will astonish you. They may criticise you to your face, write letters to journals about you, or denigrate your efforts quietly behind your back. You have to accept this if you want to continue to influence things. It should not put you off, any more than the potential for encountering road rage should stop you driving. There are ways of handling and managing these situations that are discussed in Section 4 of this book.

MIRROR MOMENT

Status, success and influence do not equal popularity: there are easier ways to be popular. Is it popularity or influence that you want? If the former, ask yourself if you are prepared to handle the unpopularity that you may encounter along with your growing influence.

Steps to success

So, given these principles as a framework, how do you start to raise your awareness and develop your influence? Here is a possible six-point plan:

1 *read*: a new journal, a key article, a book (*see* Chapter 8)
2 *write*: get a letter, article or opinion piece published in a journal (*see* Chapter 17), contact a national organisation, respond to a consultation
3 *join*: a local group, a national network, a new professional association (*see* Chapter 20)
4 *network*: locally, regionally, nationally, internationally, by phone, visit, email or internet (*see* Chapter 14)
5 *contact*: a specific individual, like-minded people, a different profession, a dissenter (*see* Chapter 23)
6 *contribute*: to a group (*see* Chapter 20), a meeting (*see* Chapter 19) or a conference (*see* Chapter 22).

PERSONAL DEVELOPMENT EXERCISE

Before you finish this book, complete all the tasks in this list:

- read a new journal regularly
- ring up someone in a different organisation to compare practice
- send your CV to somebody
- visit a department in your organisation that you have never contacted before
- arrange to shadow a board member in your organisation
- write a letter to a journal.

CHECKLIST FOR ACTION

Before you go on to the next section, check that you have completed the following:

- identified the domains of awareness that are of most interest to you
- listed your ambitions for the next year and the future.

SECTION 2

Developing awareness

CHAPTER 7

The 'well-aware' practitioner

The commonest mistake people make is trying to lead without credibility. (Helen McCloughry)

Awareness is a state of mind and a habit of behaviour rather than a finite quality that can be measurably achieved. There is never a point at which you can say 'Right, I'm aware now, what shall I do next?' Like a coin-fed electricity meter, awareness has to be constantly topped up if it is to continue to provide energy for the various activities it supports.

Top tip: *do your homework – make sure you know what you're talking about (you can only bullshit for so long!).* (Rosalynde Lowe)

The commonest mistake people make is not doing the preparatory work. (Sue Boran)

There are some characteristics that mark out the 'well-aware' practitioner:

- they know the background issues behind their area of work
- they can discuss the current 'hot topics' related to their work
- they know 'who's who' in their profession or discipline, locally and nationally
- they understand something of the wider health system in which they work
- they know where and how to find more information
- they have a range of contacts in a variety of places: they generally 'know a man who can . . .' – or a 'woman who does'!
- they are curious, questioning and prepared to put extra energy into the things they are involved in.

MIRROR MOMENT

Does this sound like you? How far do you recognise these characteristics in yourself? Think of another person who fits these characteristics: what is your instinctive reaction to them: admiration, envy, resentment?

You have to understand the context others are operating in, and their constraints – otherwise you're operating blind. (Alison Norman)

PERSONAL DEVELOPMENT EXERCISE

Fill in Table 7.1 for yourself, and your particular area of interest. This will not necessarily be the area you work in. It could be that area you identified at the end of the last section. Remember that awareness is not measurable in numerical terms so there is no overall score at the end of this exercise. It is simply intended to highlight the areas in which you already have good information and networks, and those where you could develop your awareness further. There are many other questions you could ask yourself. The table is just a starter.

TABLE 7.1 Checklist of your awareness of your area of interest

Ask yourself . . .	Score out of 5 1 = more to do, 5 = well aware	Things to do to increase score
Do I know who leads on this topic locally and nationally?		
Am I in touch with other places where they have good practice on this?		
Am I reading the right journals that cover my subject, at a range of levels?		
Are there interested people in other organisations I network with?		
Does my manager/team leader know I'm particularly interested in this?		
Where do they do good courses/who publishes good books on it?		
Are there charities or independent sector organisations I could talk to on this topic?		
Which government minister leads on this?		
What is happening to policy in this area?		
What do patients/clients/carers think are the big issues in this area?		
What changes have there been in care/treatment in the last 2 years, and what is likely to come next?		

PORTFOLIO POINTER

Use what you have learned from this exercise to identify some personal development actions and note these in your portfolio. They can form part of your continuing professional development plan.

Being a 'well-aware' practitioner

The 'well-aware' practitioner does not have a particular personality or gene that enables them to know more than other people. Nor do they need to have more time, more intelligence or a less demanding job than anyone else. There are intelligent people in key jobs who have an extraordinarily narrow perspective on the world of health and social care. And there are frantically busy practitioners who juggle home, work, hobbies and families, but still have a broad and constantly growing awareness of what is happening in the wider world. The techniques for developing awareness are available to everyone, because they depend on the use of three characteristics that are shared by everyone to some degree. These are the 'three Cs':

- curiosity
- cunning
- cheek.

Curiosity is what makes some people look up a clinical condition they have not encountered before, or ask someone to explain it. Curiosity makes people read articles on topics they don't need to know about, watch discussion programmes, go to conferences, listen to strangers talking, and accept unfamiliar tasks. It is almost the opposite of being focused, which might logically seem a prerequisite for developing awareness: it is about being eclectic, interested, and positively indiscriminate. Those nuggets of information, or ideas, or contacts that you gain as a result of exercising your curiosity, can be squirrelled away and may serve only to give you a different perspective and a broader understanding. Or they may come back months or years later to provide an essential platform for a job application, or a piece of work, which you could not have anticipated. The key principle is that nothing you do or learn is ever wasted: so the more you do and learn, the more benefit you gain. This is the toddler's approach to life: an endlessly repeated refrain of 'But why . . .?'

> TOP TIP: *build your knowledge base – be up to date, understand policy, and create informal networks. Get involved in wider agendas – professional bodies, Healthcare Commission, Audit Commission, Department of Health.*
> (FRAN WOODARD)

Exercising your natural cunning helps to ensure that you get the most and best opportunities to develop awareness, and that you make the best possible use of those opportunities when they happen. For example:

- if you offer to review books for a journal, you will get a free copy of the book to keep (and the time taken to read it can be part of your CPD activities) – *see* Chapter 8 on 'Awareness through reading'
- volunteering for a task that nobody else wants to do gives you a chance to become the local expert on that topic – in work time – as well as 'brownie points' for volunteering. *See* Chapter 15 on 'How to become an expert'
- you can choose topics for your training and development that will help you not only in your current job, but also in the one you want to get next
- if you have to find a mentor or supervisor for a piece of course work or project, asking the most prestigious and/or interesting person you can find, rather than one you know and are comfortable with, gives you a valuable new contact as well as a more challenging source of advice. *See* Chapter 11 on 'The contribution of mentors'.

The key point here is that you should set out to use every opportunity for more than one purpose: a sort of 'principle of double benefit'.

> TOP TIP: *offer to work or help outside your comfort zone . . . that way you learn more and have the opportunity to be part of different/new networks. So put yourself forward, take a chance.* (JOANNA PARKER)

Cheek is a difficult term to accept. As children we were told off for cheek, and the last thing any of us want to do is elicit responses like 'What a cheek!' from our colleagues. But cheek can mean something other than insolence and shamelessness. It is used here to mean boldness and risk taking.

Being humble, hanging back or waiting to be invited may work, but you may wait a long time for a chance to fulfil your potential. On the other hand, having the 'cheek' to send someone a copy of your project report, or ask for a high-level mentor, or ring up someone you don't know, may occasionally prove fruitless: more often it will lead to a leap forward in your awareness or your influence. But knowing how to go about it in the most effective way is essential. The rest of this book sets out to advise on applying your natural cheek in a way that gets results without giving offence: what you might call 'cheek with chic'.

To summarise, you don't need to do a taught Masters' programme or a leadership development programme to gain awareness, though these are wonderful opportunities if they come along, and can contribute enormously. The important tools for increasing awareness are natural attributes, consciously exercised and applied to the deliberate process of becoming a 'well-aware' practitioner.

CHAPTER 8

Awareness through reading

Be well informed . . . read a good-quality newspaper, gather information and data – understand it and be able to discuss it. (SUE BORAN)

Fortunately, increasing your awareness through reading is not simply a matter of reading more. Much more important than the volume of material you read is:

- what you read
- how you read it
- what you do with what you read.

It is these three elements that determine how useful your reading is in raising your awareness.

What you read

It is easy to become lazy about reading for work. We all tend to read the journals we read as students or in our early practice days, or the magazines that lie around at work, or that come to us – eventually – via the circulation list. If one comes along with membership of a professional organisation or union, then that might get a look too.

MIRROR MOMENT

Review your work-related reading. Is it as described above – or do you really seek out other useful sources of information too? How long is it since you reviewed what you read, or tried a new journal?

Widening your reading

A better approach is to explore a wider range of reading matter before fixing on those journals that give the most useful and relevant material. For instance, look at:

- other professions' journals where they work closely with your profession – for example, practice nurses read general practitioners' (GPs') journals

- care group or condition-focused journals relevant to your work or interests, rather than those addressing a particular profession – journals about stroke care, for example, rather than just physiotherapy or speech and language therapy journals
- different kinds of publication: those publishing research as well as those providing opinion and commentary; weekly magazines and monthly journals; those aimed at managers as well as at practitioners. Don't forget general newspapers that cover health and social matters intelligently and in depth.

If you do this for a few weeks, you should be able to fix on two or three that between them contain enough about the clinical, research, organisational, policy and patient perspectives on health and social care to help develop your general awareness – and in particular, the domain of awareness that you identified at the end of Section 1 for further work. It is often better to read a small number of journals regularly, getting to know the format, the writers and the main issues, and following debates from week to week, than to skim through a larger number.

Reading more widely, and exploring a large number of different publications to find some relevant new ones, does not have to involve major expense. If you are cunning (and occasionally cheeky) you can:

- borrow someone else's copy
- ask colleagues from other professions to pass on their copies
- ask a colleague to share a subscription
- suggest a subscription as a suitable use of trust, drug company or charitable funds – for the team's professional development
- read the online version for a 'taster'
- go to libraries or resource centres to look at copies
- pick up freebie copies at conferences
- organise 'journal swap' arrangements with other wards, sites or organisations.

PERSONAL DEVELOPMENT EXERCISE

Make a point of reading one new journal or other publication each week for the next three weeks, even if you already read a range of publications. There is always a chance you will find one that suits your needs better, or at least find a new perspective on a familiar topic.

Other reading

There are many sources of information: don't forget what is commonly known as the grey literature, which includes internal documents and reports, and can help further your knowledge base. (Julia Quickfall)

It is not just print publications that constitute useful reading for awareness. Don't forget to look at relevant websites: those of other professions, Royal Colleges, government departments, patient groups, lobby groups and charities. You will have a much fuller picture of your area of work and interest by seeing it from these different viewpoints. You may choose to read and respond to electronic bulletin boards, chat rooms or email groups: the quality of these varies, but they can be a really good, almost real-time opportunity to share information, develop views and make contact with people who share your clinical or work interests.

How to read

The first trick is not to let the journals or other reading pile up for weeks – the guilt factor is worse than finding the time to read them in the week they arrive. It also means that you will miss the moment to respond to a letter or article, or a conversation string in an email group.

Make a point of reading everything in the publication: not just the main articles, but the news, analysis, opinions and letters. They all provide a broader view of the subject area. Note the kinds of people who write for each journal and where they work: they could be worth contacting to compare notes on shared areas of work, or ask for more information.

Whether reading a publication, a website or an email string, make a deliberate effort to relate what you are reading to your own situation, rather than simply taking it in as interesting information. Ask yourself:

- do we do that?
- should we change what we do, or should they?
- do we have anything to contribute to their knowledge or practice?
- how does this compare with my experience?

Look out for opportunities to start to influence people: letters you could respond to, award competitions you could enter, consultations you could respond to or campaigns you might support.

What to do with what you read

The first step is take up those opportunities you have identified – quickly! Generally, the longer you wait and think about it, the less likely you are to get round to writing that letter, or downloading the consultation document, or emailing the new contact. So do it as soon as possible – taking just enough time to make sure you do it well, of course (*see* Chapter 23 on writing letters and emails, for example). Also:

- keep a file or box of particularly relevant articles, and/or a list of references to ensure you can find them again – it avoids those moments when you say 'I read somewhere that . . .' but can't substantiate it.
- have an organised way of noting contact names, with relevant details so that you know why you noted down the name in the first place. It doesn't matter whether it's a diary, address book, personal organiser or computer – but you will need your network of contacts to be accessible, legible and comprehensible, if you are to benefit from having them.

PERSONAL DEVELOPMENT EXERCISE

Find one new or interesting fact or opinion in this week's journal, and follow it up. Make contact with the author, or write in to comment on it yourself. File the article for future reference.

CHECKLIST FOR ACTION

Have you:

- tried out some new journals?
- looked at some relevant websites?
- decided what publications you will read regularly, and sorted out how you will access them?

CHAPTER 9

Clinical awareness

The commonest mistake people make is not communicating with all involved – many forget that the most important people you need on side are the clerical staff and assistants, not just the clinicians and managers.
(SANDRA MELLORS)

Clinical awareness is a subset of awareness: it is awareness of physical states or conditions, how those conditions affect people, and how they are best treated and cared for. It is not only for people working in 'hands-on' clinical jobs, like clinical scientists, therapists or midwives: it is just as important for others working in the same service to have a well-developed awareness of clinical matters, if they are to influence effectively. It is a matter of knowing the business you are in, whatever your role.

I have found over the years since I left 'clinical practice' (i.e. working directly 'hands on' with patients) that there can be a degree of snobbery about things clinical. People who are in clinical roles can be very dismissive of anyone who works in a different role, no matter how significant, in the health service. 'But with respect . . .' (which means the opposite) they sometimes say to the 'non-clinician', 'How long is it since you worked *clinically* . . .?' If the question is addressed at a long-time manager who is about to perform a delicate clinical task, it might be legitimate. But if it just aimed at making the non-clinician feel inadequate, it isn't. It fails to recognise that there is expertise and experience in all roles that may be very relevant to the situation in hand, and should be respected.

MIRROR MOMENT

Think for a moment about your reaction to the words 'clinical', 'hands on' and 'frontline', as applied to people who work directly with patients. Do these terms feel complimentary or derogatory to you? How do you use them? Do you genuinely believe that all kinds of expertise and experience are equally valuable to the interests of the patient?

Of course, prejudices always work both ways, and there are just as many managers, educators and others who regard working directly with patients or clients as the lowest rung of the health service ladder, to be left as soon as possible on the way up.

Exploring clinical awareness

So what could clinical awareness consist of? At individual level, it is focused on the clinical condition of the patient, and radiates outward from that to encompass a whole range of different aspects (*see* Figure 9.1) including for example:

- *the condition*: which might be a disease, a syndrome, or a biological state such as old age, or pregnancy
- *the expression of that condition for the individual*: the signs and symptoms, the chemical, physical or biological indicators, the changes that can be measured or felt
- *the treatment and care required*: the kind, length and success of treatment, the supporting services required, the availability of appropriate care and services, the developments imminent or anticipated through research and development
- *the impact on the individual, their family and society*: in terms of changes to capacity and independence, pain, disability (temporary or permanent), spread to others, need for care, support and treatment, etc
- *the background to the condition*: how widespread it is, what its origins are, what is known and not known about it . . .

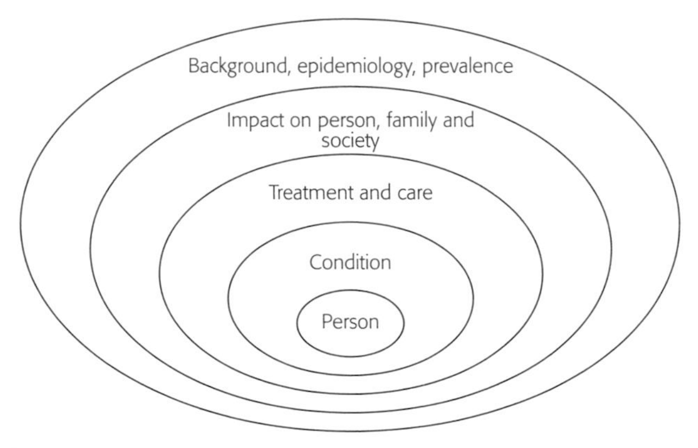

Figure 9.1 Clinical awareness

> *It's a mistake to be a 'single issue' person, not seeing the big picture.* (ALISON NORMAN)

It is easy, particularly when life is very busy, to focus in on the condition, and the more obvious aspects of its expression, or on one individual patient, and not look much further. This is the approach often caricatured as talking about 'the hysterectomy in the sideward' or 'doing the diabetics'. However, the real problem with such a narrow approach is that it leads to two opposite, and equally unhelpful, modes of behaviour that get in the way of influencing change:

- *condition-myopia*: which occurs when someone is a real technical expert on the detail of the condition in question, but completely fails to see the wider context. So, for example, they try to persuade their trust to print a comprehensive patient information leaflet on a condition that is so rare that the trust is unlikely to see another one for a decade, or so complex that sufferers are not treated at the trust anyway. When they fail to do so, they consider themselves to be powerless to influence – rather than thinking they may have been pursuing the wrong avenue of influence
- *individual-fixation*: this is perhaps the single problem which causes the most obstacles to influence – a health worker being so completely focused on patients as individuals that they cannot appreciate the wider picture in relation to the condition. So, for example, they write to their MP demanding a change in immunisation policy based on their experiences with a handful of individuals, without looking at the wider picture of evidence, research and public health factors.

The ideal of clinical awareness would be taking a slice out of the 'cake' in Figure 9.1 for each patient, client or family, and making a deliberate effort to see the whole picture, from condition to background.

But what activities or behaviours can a busy health worker realistically expect to include in their practice on a regular basis to develop this sort of awareness? You could try:

- looking up a familiar diagnostic label in a dictionary, to check that your use of the terminology is accurate and up to date (is it 'juvenile onset diabetes' or 'type 1 diabetes' or 'insulin-dependent diabetes' these days?)
- checking for normal values of relevant blood and other tests, and the exact diagnostic threshold for the condition (what level of hyperglycaemia is diagnostic of diabetes? Who says so?)
- asking other members of the team (medical, technical, therapy), about latest developments in knowledge, care and treatment from their professional perspective
- reading about the condition in sources you would not normally read: instead of just your usual journals, try the internet, or newsletters from patients' groups, or the autobiography of someone who has the condition (such as Sir Steven Redgrave, the Olympic rower, in the case of diabetes)
- visiting another ward, unit or clinic where the same, or related, conditions are treated, to get a different perspective (if you work in a hospital metabolic unit, go to see how newly diagnosed diabetic patients are stabilised on insulin in their own homes – or vice versa)
- looking up a relevant patient support group or charity on the internet, such as Diabetes UK, to see what help, information and support is provided from non-statutory sources.

PERSONAL DEVELOPMENT EXERCISE

Do all of the above for one condition this month. Make a note of anything you learn in your personal professional profile, together with a follow-up plan: reversing the 'job shadowing', sharing the information with your team, or getting a copy of the authoritative guidelines.

Using available resources

It will be clear from this exercise that developing and maintaining clinical awareness means using all the resources available to you. Wherever you work, and whatever your role, you should have access to colleagues, books, journals and, just as importantly, patients, their families and carers. No-one is without resources for developing this awareness. In some posts, or at home, you may also have access to the internet, including e-discussion groups, websites of relevant charities and lobby groups, and links to policy documents, guidelines, and information from other countries. Within the NHS, similar (or contrasting) wards, units or clinics are only a phone call away, and site visits are a valid part of professional development. Time, of course, is the resource most often cited as an obstacle to these sorts of activities. But many of them – like asking a colleague a question, or visiting a website – can take very little time.

Well-developed awareness is essential for influence. Remember the three Cs:

- *cunning*: a little flattery can get you a lot of free education – experts from all professions like to share their knowledge and demonstrate their skills. Ask and you shall receive, and most of it during your 'day job'
- *curiosity*: ask that question, or click on that hypertext link – nothing you find is wasted, even if it doesn't contribute to solving today's problem
- *cheek*: phone up the author of an article, suggest a journal swap with a colleague from another profession, ask if you can attend a patients' group meeting. You may occasionally be rebuffed, but more often you will learn something useful, and build up your network of contacts at the same time.

Be alive to, and develop your understanding of, the direction in which your service is going, and what the wider positive and negative influences are.
(Sue Norman)

CHECKLIST FOR ACTION

Before you go on to the next chapter, have you:

- learned something new about a familiar condition?
- recorded your investigations in your portfolio?
- written a follow-up action plan?

CHAPTER 10

Making the most of conferences and events

Many conferences are a waste of time and money that could be better spent on a mentor or coach. (ROSALYNDE LOWE)

This chapter focuses specifically on the big regional or national conferences, but many of the suggestions within it would apply equally to study days and workshops. There are, however, real differences in outlook and atmosphere, as well as scale, from a big national conference, and they offer unparalleled opportunities. Only at the big conferences can you regularly expect to:

- hear politicians speak, announce new policies and answer questions from the floor
- listen to and question the leaders of health or professional organisations, unions and statutory bodies in workshop settings
- meet the people whose names you read in the journals
- meet journal editors and book publishers
- hear about the latest ideas and research
- see the latest products relevant to your area of work
- pick up policy documents, buy discounted books and get free copies of magazines and journals
- meet lots of other professionals from similar areas of work, and exchange ideas and contacts.

So it is definitely worth making every effort to attend at least one major conference a year. As well as providing professional development, a couple of days at a conference can be a well-deserved break from the daily round. The chance to focus on your topic, to learn something new, listen to debate and see your work from a different perspective, is a rare luxury.

Remember we always learn something at conferences, even if we know the subject matter inside out. (BARBARA STUTTLE)

The big stumbling block of course is the cost. The conference can cost a few hundred pounds – though some are cheaper – and then there is accommodation and travel to fund as well. Time out from work can be another problem, depending on your employer and the demands of the service. Once you have chosen the conference that you are determined to attend (*see* below on finding the right conference), then the ruthless application of cunning and cheek can sometimes solve the resource problem. Try:

- submitting a paper or poster to the conference (*see* Chapter 22) so that all your expenses are paid by the organisers – but look out for the few conferences (usually the international ones) which still expect speakers to pay
- offering to run a workshop at the conference – again, expenses paid
- offering to put on a local study day afterwards to pass on key messages, cascade information or demonstrate new equipment, to persuade your employer to pay for the conference
- identifying the item on the programme of most relevance to your area of work, or the key expert speaker, and suggest you write up their session for dissemination round your unit, for the same purpose
- sharing the cost with your employer
- accessing any charitable trust funds, grants or gift monies available locally for professional development
- applying for national training or development bursaries or awards
- offering to pay for travel, or accommodation expenses, as your contribution – then look for nearby relatives to stay with, and cheap deals on rail tickets
- as a last resort (which many people use) take annual leave and pay for yourself.

Remember that you have to invest in yourself – effort, time and sometimes money too – if you want to be in a position to have real influence.

Choosing the right conference

> *Before you even pay your conference fee and block out the time in your diary, think carefully about why you want to go, what you want to achieve, and what the ideal outcome will be for you.* (Rosalynde Lowe)

Given the difficulty of finding time and funding, choosing the right conference is very important. Information about conferences can be found in the professional journals – which often have double page spreads listing the whole conference programme – or in the separate conference 'flyers' which are inserted into journals, pinned up on notice boards or available in the library or online.

> *Be seen at appropriate events – for exposure.* (Fran Woodard)

The key is to be fussy and make a positive decision for positive reasons, not negative reasons (*see* Box 10.1). It is rather like booking a holiday: you wouldn't go somewhere without comparing brochures, checking value for money, knowing something about the amenities and the attractions on offer and feeling excited by the prospect. So

– unless you are 'sent' to a conference with absolutely no choice – here are some key questions to consider.

What do you want from the conference?

- Is it to hear original research papers, or to hear from people engaged in a particular area of clinical practice? They may be at different conferences.
- Is it to meet like-minded colleagues and exchange views, pick up information and debate current issues? Then you want a conference with debates, question and answer sessions, an exhibition, small group workshops, fringe meetings and so on.
- Is it to tell policy makers and politicians that they have got it wrong, and argue for more money, less interference or a different approach? Then you need a conference with a government minister or official attending, a questions session, debate and, preferably, voting, and high-profile media coverage.

What sort of people do you want to hear from?

> *Use all the breaks to network, but find out in advance who are the people you need to talk to and target them.* (Sandra Mellors)

Do you want to hear from politicians and Department of Health or Work and Pensions officials, or people in practice? Researchers, clinicians, professional advisors or educationalists? Leading-edge practitioners, or mainstream people in 'ordinary' jobs? Or a mixture of these? Every conference will have a different mix of speakers and presenters, so the conference programme bears close scrutiny. Look out for:

- 'to be confirmed' after a speaker's name: some conference organisers publish a 'wish list' programme, and the people you actually hear on the day may not be any of those on the original programme
- job titles and places of work alongside speakers' names: do these suggest that they are the kind of people you want to hear from? Is the person a known expert on the subject, or just someone willing to speak? Do they work in the NHS or social care – or are they management consultants?
- familiar and unfamiliar names: some people always talk on the same topic – this could make them an authoritative expert, or a bore. Their job title and the title of their presentation will help you judge if they might have something new or relevant to say. Conversely, don't be put off if you don't know any of the names: judge by their job and their topic whether they might have a fresh new perspective, or an interesting project to talk about. The best programme will bring together a mixture of familiar and unfamiliar people.

What do you want to hear about?

If it is technical, specialist or practical information, look for experts, workshop sessions and detailed, descriptive titles for papers. If it is policy, developments and the future of the health service, look for ministers, officials and professional leaders, and challenging, visionary titles. If it is practice developments, look for practising clinicians describing their projects, innovations or research.

Of course, life is rarely sufficiently neat and orderly for you to find exactly what you want on a single conference programme. It is no bad thing to take pot luck with some elements of a programme, making the most of them when you get there. Factors such as distance to travel, time of year, cost and convenience may play a part in deciding which conference you attend, alongside professional considerations. Whatever the conference, it is vital that you make the most of the opportunities it offers for expanding your awareness and enhancing your practice.

BOX 10.1 Choosing a conference

Don't go because:

- you always go to this conference
- your friend goes to this one
- it is 'the' conference for your occupational group
- the sessions are on familiar/favourite topics
- it's the cheapest you've seen.
- the title interests you
- it's in a town you'd like to visit.

Do go because:

- the speakers are worth hearing
- there will be opportunities to meet and speak to the presenters
- the programmed sessions are relevant to your work
- you will learn something new
- the format allows interaction with speakers
- there is a good range of useful stands at the exhibition
- it is aimed at attracting the kind of people it would be useful for you to meet.

MIRROR MOMENT

Stop and think about the last conference or workshop you attended. What were the most important factors in deciding your attendance? How did you attempt to influence them, and what success did you have? What did you learn from that experience that you could use to influence future opportunities for professional development?

PERSONAL DEVELOPMENT EXERCISE

Having considered these questions, write down your objectives for the next conference you attend in a few sentences. Then you can check them against what is on offer when you see a conference advertised.

Making the most of a conference

It seems obvious that, having found the time, money and opportunity to attend a conference, you should go determined to wring every ounce of benefit from it. But there is a long list of bad habits that people fall in to with regard to conferences, and that should be avoided (some are listed in Box 10.2). Everyone commits the occasional transgression, and sometimes minor rebellion can be good for the soul, but in general – and particularly if someone else is paying – you ought to plan to make the best possible use of your time at the conference.

BOX 10.2 Bad habits at a conference

- Attending only the easiest, most predictable sessions
- Relying on the handouts rather than adding your own notes
- Spending breaks alone rather than mixing
- Sticking with people you know
- Going to the exhibition just to pick up freebies
- Skipping sessions to go shopping
- Leaving early

Planning for successful conference attendance starts with the arrival of your confirmation of booking, and the conference pack or papers, if they are sent out before the conference. Check the confirmation letter to see that all details are correct, rather than just filing it: it is very embarrassing to arrive and find they have you down for the wrong day, or that they expect you to pay when you have negotiated a guest ticket. The conference papers may include:

- the entry tickets, meal and car park vouchers, workshop allocations etc that will ensure that you can gain access to the conference and the relevant sessions on arrival. Check that you have everything you asked for, as sorting it out on the day with several hundred other people in the queue at the registration desk is a nightmare
- accommodation details, if you are staying overnight. Again, double check well in advance that you are booked in where and for as long as expected, and that you have a map to find the town, the conference venue and the accommodation. If you are travelling by public transport, check on the map to find out exactly where the accommodation is. Sometimes it is well outside the town centre where the train station is, and you will need plenty of cash for a taxi, or information on buses

- the finalised programme for the event. Check that the speakers you were expecting will be there, and all the workshops are running – they are sometimes cancelled late in the run-up to the conference if they are under-booked. If you have been re-allocated to a different workshop because of a cancellation, check that you are happy with the second choice, and if not, contact the organisers. Don't worry about being a nuisance: you have after all paid a goodly fee to attend the conference. It is also more convenient for the organisers to swap your workshop choice in advance, than have unexpected people turn up on the day, unbalancing the numbers and confusing the workshop leader!

Finally, check that the venue hasn't changed: I have known people go to the wrong hotel for a conference because they didn't notice the change.

With papers in order, and any changes confirmed with the organisers, you can scrutinise the programme and begin to plan your day or days at the conference.

Look at the exhibition floor plan (if there is one) or exhibitors' list and mark the exhibitors you particularly want to visit: whether manufacturers of clinical products, support or special interest groups, professional organisations or publishers. It is easy to miss a stand, or even a whole section of a large exhibition, if you wander round vaguely on the day.

Read the speakers' biographies, often included with conference papers. Apart from helping you judge the interest and relevance of their topic, they provide little vignettes of career paths, telling you how they arrived at their current post, and why they have been invited to speak at the event. Mark those speakers you would like to talk to, ask questions of, or simply obtain a contact number for.

Write down any particular pieces of information, or resources such as samples, literature or contacts that you want to obtain. This will help you assess afterwards whether the conference has been useful, and give you specific objectives for the time you are there.

Prepare any questions you might want to ask, if there is a question and answer session (but *see* Chapter 22 for effective ways to influence at conferences).

Put some of your business cards into your conference pack, or if you don't have them, prepare some slips with your own contact details on them, so that you can give them to people you meet at the conference.

At the conference

> *Network like mad, gather information and talk to people – you might find out interesting and useful things.* (Deb Lapthorne)

A practical tip is to wear your delegate name badge high up in the area of your collar bone, not half way down your chest or on your belt. This makes it much easier for people to note your name and organisation, and start a conversation. Equally, it helps people you have impressed with your conversation to remember you.

Make the most of the speakers' sessions by making brief notes during the session, and collecting any copies of presentations or background information that are not already in your conference pack. Look out for lessons you can learn from their way of presenting, for when you are doing conference presentations. What works well in their manner, their appearance, their use of formal and informal material, their use of notes and slides? What irritates you about their style – mannerisms, body language, use of material, tone?

> *Ask questions of speakers: if you are interested in making quite sure they know who you are, go and speak with them after the presentation. Leave them your business card.* (SUE NORMAN)

After the speaker has finished, consider whether it would be useful to meet them, to comment immediately, or to obtain contact details for later. If they are the last speaker before a break, they will probably be available at the front of the auditorium for a few minutes after their session has ended. Speakers are almost always happy to be approached, and to discuss what they have said. After all, they would not have agreed to give a presentation if they were cripplingly shy or modest. Starting with a positive or at least neutral statement – 'I really enjoyed your talk' or 'That was very interesting' – provides a better platform for discussion than 'What a load of rubbish that was', however strongly you might feel about it. In this setting there is rarely much time, so it is usually best to use the moment to establish your interest, and suggest a contact later. 'We are doing a similar project, but taking a multidisciplinary approach' or 'I've just done a literature search on this, and there are some studies that show very different results from yours' can be followed by the offer of your business card or contact slip, and the promise to ring or email in the next couple of weeks. This sort of approach to speakers is common, so don't hesitate to make the first move. It can be the start not only of a fruitful network, but also of becoming more widely known in your area of expertise: an essential first step towards developing real influence.

> *Be brave – never regret not asking a question or making your point (even if you have to approach speakers in the breaks).* (JUDITH ELLIS)

If the speaker is not immediately available, note the name and the face, and jot down the point you want to make to them. Then you can catch them at the end of the full session.

Some speakers – such as government ministers – are not likely to be approachable after a speech, as they are usually whisked away to their next engagement, or to meet the local VIPs. Often the only chance to make a point to a minister – and an additional opportunity with other speakers – is through a question and answer session.

Questions and answers

It was suggested earlier that you note down any questions you might want to ask before arriving at the conference. The essential corollary to this is that you are prepared to amend or abandon the question if it is answered in the course of the presentation. Nothing sounds quite so contrived and embarrassing as a questioner standing up to demand to know something that they have just been told, or to make a rabble-rousing speech. If, however, your question is still relevant, or the presentation has raised a new question in your mind, then *do*:

- jot it down as coherently as you can while the preliminaries are still underway, or another questioner has the microphone
- indicate clearly to the chair that you have a question: raise your hand fully, or stand up, or whatever you have been invited to do. A hesitant half wave is unlikely to be successful – remember, half the audience is yawning, stretching and twitching at this point
- wait for the 'roving mike', if there is one, and use it properly (*see* Box 10.3). If not, keep your head up (lift your notes up to read them, rather than ducking your head) and speak loudly and clearly, directly to the person who will answer the question
- start pleasantly, even if you have a razor sharp question and intend to use it. A simple 'good morning' or 'thank you for speaking so openly' inclines the speaker to give your question sympathetic consideration
- be professional in your manner. A long preamble explaining your local situation, or rabble-rousing the audience around you, makes it very difficult for the speaker to pick out the actual question you want answered
- ask only one thing. Not, for example, 'So can you tell us why that money seems to have disappeared, and how we are supposed to change services when you don't even have a proper definition of what "intermediate care" actually is – our trust says the money isn't ring fenced so it's probably gone on other things, and is that right? We'd like to know how to access the money for training and how much is really being spent on health services and how much is going to social services'. There are at least six different questions in there, and you would be lucky to get a specific answer to even one of them. A rambling question usually elicits a rambling answer, and no-one is satisfied.

BOX 10.3 Need to know: how to use a hand-held microphone

- Wait for it to arrive.
- Check with the person who hands it over if it is already switched on.
- Hold it close to your mouth and don't let it sink away as you speak.
- Keep your head still while speaking: if you look round, it cannot pick up your voice.
- Keep it away from jewellery or buttons that will rattle at high volume.
- If you keep hold of it while listening to the answer, keep it still and don't put it down or in your lap while it is still on.
- If you get a loud feedback screech, don't panic – the audiovisual technician will sort it out.
- Remember that it will pick up any snorts, sniggers or expletives that slip out while you have it in your hand!

Some question and answer sessions descend into highly unsatisfactory and acrimonious grumbles, in spite of the best efforts of the chair, if questioners or audience misbehave. So *don't*:

- be gratuitously offensive or insulting to the speakers
- discuss the questions or answers with your neighbours during the session
- hang on to the microphone and try to engage in a dialogue with the speaker
- deliberately provoke the audience into noisy unrest – you may get a round of applause for a succinct and pointed question, but this is quite different from setting off a series of muttered discussions while the speaker is trying to hear your question
- spend the time packing your bag, arranging rendezvous with your colleagues and sneaking out to get into the lunch queue.

Making the most of the exhibition

> *Decide to talk to at least three people you have never met before at each break during the conference programme.* (Joanna Parker)

Most medium and large national conferences have some sort of exhibition attached. There is usually some time built into the programme for delegates to look round the exhibition, though some people use it to have an extra cup of coffee, to go shopping in the town or head back to their hotel. But the exhibition can be an extremely useful opportunity to meet three basic conference objectives:

- to make new contacts
- to pick up useful information
- to meet key people.

Contacts

Many major nursing organisations, statutory bodies, nursing journals and publishers have stands at major conferences. There are also product manufacturers, voluntary and patient organisations, charities and representatives of trusts. Their editors, professional advisors, education and professional officers and others are often available on the stand, and this is an excellent opportunity to talk to them about your work or professional interests, or about writing an article. Make sure you leave your contact details following a fruitful discussion, and take the details of the individual you were talking to. It is far easier and more effective to write later to a named individual whom you have met, rather than addressing a letter impersonally.

Information

Most big conferences provide you with a bag of some sort for your conference information. Discard the flyers, adverts and other detritus (after a quick perusal to check if you actually want it), and use the bag for some of the genuinely useful items you can pick up from the exhibition. Take, for example:

- issues of journals you don't usually read, to see if you might want to subscribe, read them or write for them in future

- copies of professional guidance that you never quite get round to ordering in the day to day rush – from your professional regulator, union or specialist association
- copies of Department of Health guidance or policy documents that would take months to reach you on circulation at work
- literature from manufacturers on new drugs, or products, or equipment
- publishers' catalogues of healthcare titles
- lists of useful website addresses, voluntary organisations, or other composite material.

Key people

The exhibition is often your best opportunity to buttonhole key people from the unions, professional organisations or Department of Health. While you may not get all the answers you want, it is a chance to make an impression, highlight an important issue, and give them your contact details. If you are interested in shadowing or secondment experience, ask if you can send them your CV. If you have a particular project or achievement you want to publicise, offer to send them a summary. If you want to champion a pet cause, ask their advice on other contacts or networks relevant to the topic. Providing you are polite and professional in your approach, it cannot do any harm, and it may well reap results, if not shortly, then in the longer-term. The key thing to remember is that this is an investment in your future: however difficult it feels to push yourself forward in this way, it is expected, it is common and it is effective.

After the event

As ever, it is important to reflect on and record what you have gained from attending the conference. The summary of learning, together with the conference programme, handouts and other materials, belongs in your professional portfolio. This is also the place to record what changes you made in your practice resulting from this learning.

A summary of key information should also go to your employer and whoever funded your attendance at the conference. This could be as short as a few bullet points, and may not even be expected: in this case, it only underlines your professionalism and initiative! If you promised to put on a study day, or talk to a meeting about the conference, do it sooner rather than later, even though you are immediately drowning in work again. It doesn't get any easier with time, so you might as well do it while it is fresh in your mind.

Keep any promises made at the conference. If you offered to send out a CV, or project summary, or idea for an article, do it within a couple of weeks – and the sooner the better. If you said you would ring someone to talk about your work, try to fit that in earlier rather than later. The longer it lapses, the less likely you are to believe that they will remember you and want to hear from you.

Think about next time: look back at the programme, the papers and the workshops, and ask yourself what you could have contributed to the conference. You will have been aware that some of the speakers were 'first timers': could that be you next year?

PERSONAL DEVELOPMENT EXERCISE

Look at as many conference flyers relevant to your area of work as you can find, on notice boards, websites, or in journals. Practise appraising the information on them to see how relevant the conference would be to meeting your identified CPD objectives. Whether or not you can find funding for any of them, it is good to practise the skills needed to select the most appropriate events.

CHECKLIST FOR ACTION

Before going on to the next chapter, have you:

- listed some objectives for the next conference you will attend?
- assessed a number of conference programmes to judge which will best meet your stated objectives?

CHAPTER 11

The contribution of mentors

> *How else would you get the undivided attention and problem-solving ability of a senior and experienced person?* (Deb Lapthorne)

If you want to increase your awareness of the world of health and social care generally, or your specialism or service in particular, it makes sense to use not only your own resources, but those available from other people too. While professional reading and attending conferences or workshops are activities that you can do alone, there are other professional development opportunities that are only effective when you share your hopes and ambitions with someone else.

'Mentor' is defined in an ordinary dictionary as 'an experienced and trusted advisor', and 'mentorship' in a nursing dictionary as 'a system which provides support to students during their training'. Somewhere between the two lies the current trend for many professionals – not only students – to meet regularly with a more experienced practitioner who has agreed to be their mentor. In fact, and in common with other such developments, there seems to be a view that you can't have too much of a good thing, and some people have two mentors, for different aspects of their practice and career. Sometimes one is from the same and one from a different profession. What they will have in common is a commitment to give their time and the benefit of their experience to assist the 'mentee'. Other forms of professional support, such as a preceptorship and clinical supervision, have different characteristics to mentorship – *see* the 'need to know' information in Box 11.1.

BOX 11.1 Need to know: different kinds of professional support

- *Mentorship* is usually used to mean a series of one-to-one meetings with someone (or more than one person on different occasions) working in your field, who is more senior or more experienced than you. This person has agreed formally to meet with you in order to help you address specific personal development and workplace issues. The arrangement may be for a defined length of time, and involve agreement on the frequency, nature and purpose of meetings.
- *Clinical supervision* is a process designed to provide time and opportunity to reflect on your practice. It may take place in a one-to-one meeting with a supervisor, or in a

group with peers. In some health and social care professions (including midwifery and psychology) it is mandatory, and systems for supervision are well established. In others (such as nursing) it remains voluntary, and takes place in a variety of ways.

- *Preceptorship* is the support given to newly qualified practitioners for a defined length of time – often six months or a year – after qualification. It usually involves some degree of informal support and oversight by a named person in the same workplace.
- *Coaching* is similar to mentorship in being a negotiated, one-to-one relationship aimed at helping an individual find their own solutions and strategies for success in their job and their career – and the terms are sometimes used interchangeably. However a coach is less likely to be someone from the same profession as the person they are coaching, and more likely to be from outside of health and social care altogether. People are more likely to have to pay for coaching.

Much has been written about the mentor–mentee relationship, and the nature and scope of the transactions between them. But in simple terms, the role of the mentor could be described as:

- a sounding board for the rehearsal of issues, concerns, successes and dilemmas
- a mirror, reflecting back the situation or concern in a different light
- a challenger, making the mentee unpick situations, and find their own solutions or approaches
- a signpost to information, contacts, and different perspectives.

A mentor is not meant to be a protector, problem solver, best friend, or shortcut to promotion. Meetings with a mentor are not necessarily easy, but the gains in personal and career development are worth the effort that should go into the dialogue between mentor and mentee.

> *The more senior the post you are in, the more difficult it is to share concerns and difficulties. Having a safe place to discuss issues is, from my own experience, vital.* (SUE NORMAN)

Why a mentor?

> *Mentors are an absolute must even if you have a good supervisor or manager: one-to-ones will always be taken up with the business need – you need reflective space.* (SUZANNE HILTON)

Most people who have a mentor would agree that they have two objectives for the relationship: developing themselves in their practice, and furthering their career. For this reason, they often choose as a mentor someone in a post they would like to be occupying in the future, or who has the qualities they consider they need to acquire their ultimate job. In this case, the mentor is like a role model with dialogue. The mentor does not have to be in the same organisation, and the perspective offered by a cross-organisational partnership can be particularly useful. So, if you work in primary care, consider a mentor from an acute setting – but one who understands the wider system. If you work in a trust, consider a mentor from a different kind of organisation. This helps to focus discussions on the real, underlying issues and dilemmas, rather than obscuring them behind your common experience of organisational structures or personalities.

> *Don't go for the obvious person to be your mentor, mentors from outside your current sphere of work or influence can offer fresh insights.* (Joanna Parker)

A mentor does not necessarily have to be geographically close, as some mentorship relationships work very satisfactorily by a combination of face-to-face and telephone contact. Alternatively, individuals can travel out of their area and 'meet in the middle', with the advantages of freedom from interruptions, a neutral setting and a very real sense of having left the daily round behind.

The key is to be clear what you want from your mentor, and so what kind of person they need to be in terms of post, experience and approach.

MIRROR MOMENT

Think about what you would want from a mentor: don't have anyone in mind at this point, but try to take a purely objective view. What would help you to gain confidence, cope better at work, take the next step towards your goals – or clarify your career goals? Then think what kind of person might provide this.

Finding a mentor

> *A mentor is enormously helpful if you get the right one, not so helpful if you get one that is only ever positive and can't deal with difficult stuff, so shop around and ask several people about their experience before deciding.* (Deb Lapthorne)

With a clear view of the kind of person you are looking for, you can look around locally, regionally or nationally to find someone whom you think could help you. It is also worth asking other people for suggestions – they may have people in their network of contacts who would be ideal. It is not necessary to know someone before they become a mentor: remember this is a business relationship rather than a friendship, though the latter may well develop over time.

> *You will need different types of mentors at different times. I tend to alternate between 'cuddly and supportive' types and 'hard-edged challenging' people.* (Helen Mould)

Having identified a potential mentor, the best way to approach them is probably by email, if you don't know them well, or in person if you already meet with them. Be prepared to say:

- why you feel you need mentorship
- what you hope to achieve from the relationship
- that you are prepared to commit to an agreed trial period for the mentorship
- that you have discussed and agreed the idea with your manager, if you intend to pursue the mentorship during your working hours.

> *You should refresh and replace the relationship over time as need changes.*
> (Fran Woodard)

As the mentoring relationship means a regular commitment of time, energy and effort on both sides, you can only ask – not expect – that the person you have identified will become your mentor. They may decline if they do not have the time, or if they have a number of other mentees already. This should not be seen as a personal rejection: they should be able to tell you why they cannot take on the mentorship. They may also be able to suggest someone in a similar position to themselves who might be able to become a mentor. This may or may not work: thank them for the suggestion, but make your own judgement as to whether the individual suggested can offer you the kind of experience you want.

Sometimes mentors are allocated – or can be chosen from a limited list – specifically to help develop an individual undertaking a post-registration course, or leadership programme. If such an opportunity is offered, it is worth taking, if only to explore the possibilities of mentorship. It is not essential to find the ideal mentor first time, and although such allocation may seem second best to a free choice, the individuals on the list should have been primed with information about the course, and the objectives of it, and therefore be all the more helpful.

Working with a mentor

The key to mentorship is commitment. This means:

- agreeing to meet at regular intervals for a specified period of time
- keeping to that agreement, and prioritising mentorship meetings over other calls on your time
- protecting the time from interruptions on the day
- participating fully in the mentoring: talking, listening, exploring and accepting challenges and opportunities, with the focus on your current role, professional development and career
- being fair to your mentor: building a mutually respectful and balanced relationship, and not expecting your mentor to take the blame for any failures or disappointments, or to find solutions to your problems
- sticking to the ground rules agreed at the beginning of your work together, about issues such as confidentiality, frequency of meetings, contact between meetings, and agreed endpoints or review points for the relationship.

Mentors frequently provide their mentees with very practical benefits as well as the chance for discussion and reflection. These commonly include:

- access to their own professional networks and contacts
- opportunities for job swaps, or to shadow key individuals who can provide relevant experience, or a different perspective on practice
- direction to literature, projects, individuals or sites which provide new ideas or examples for the mentee's work.

> *Before a session, give some thought to what you'd like to cover, and be prepared for the discussion to go off at a tangent – great insights come from tangents.* (ROSALYNDE LOWE)

There is no doubt that having a mentor can enhance professional development at any stage of a career. It is of course an ideal way to raise your awareness, as by definition your mentor is more experienced, with a different perspective on healthcare. It is easy to focus constantly on your current busy job, and develop a narrow view of the world of healthcare. Mentors are guaranteed to help you look up and around, an essential precursor to developing influence.

> *The contribution of mentors is essential – not all the time and not always the same one, but worthwhile especially when self-doubt creeps in!* (JUDITH WHITTAM)

Role models

Whether or not you have a mentor, most people have had one or more role models during their career. It may be someone in the same organisation, or someone you have never met, but whose career and work you have followed and admired. The difference between a role model and a mentor is of course the explicit, developmental nature of the relationship, and regularly scheduled contact, with the latter. You may never be in the same room as your role models! But they can still be a significant influence on your professional development.

There are three main kinds of behaviour that people adopt in relation to their role models, which I think of as 'mirroring', 'mimicking' and 'modelling'.

- '*Mirroring*' is when someone quite clearly copies the role model's mannerisms, figures of speech, manner of dress and way of working. They wear the same kind of suits, treat their colleagues the same way, and read the same books and journals. This is often obvious to other people around them, though it may be unconscious to some degree on the part of the admirer. In time, such close copying usually wanes as other influences come into play. It can be helpful to build confidence and establish good habits (provided the role model has good habits to be copied!), but in the longer-term, it is better to develop your own style of working rather than to try to become someone else.
- '*Mimicking*' is a more selective copying of certain traits or habits that are admired

in the role model: such as using particular terminology, or tackling problem issues in the same way. Picking and choosing like this allows you to combine the best traits of a number of role models with your own unique personality, and is more likely to be sustainable in the long-term than mirroring.
- '*Modelling*' is more general even than mimicking, and is more about absorbing the role model's attitudes and approaches than copying any particular trait.

Most people will recognise that they use a combination of these strategies in relation to many different influential people throughout their career. What is important is to be open to influence, and prepared to adopt and adapt the best characteristics of the many admirable people you will meet over the years.

PERSONAL DEVELOPMENT EXERCISE

Think of two people whose work you have admired at any stage of your working life, and whom you regard as role models for you. Try to identify those characteristics that you most admired in them or their practice. Have you incorporated those characteristics into your own work? Try to consciously demonstrate those admired characteristics in your current role in the next few days.

CHECKLIST FOR ACTION

Have you:
- written down what you want to get from a mentoring relationship?
- identified someone who you will approach to be a mentor?
- decided what admired behaviours or characteristics you will consciously use in the next few days?

CHAPTER 12

E-awareness

One of the most important factors in my career has been being IT literate.
(HELEN MCCLOUGHRY)

E-awareness – or awareness of all things electronic and computer-related, from emails to word processing and web searching – lies along such a wide spectrum that it is impossible to find a common point at which to start to discuss it. There are health professionals who lead national information technology projects setting up systems to support clinical services, and others who refuse to have anything to do with computers. There are those with daily experience of inputting clinical data into computers, and others who don't have even have regular access to a computer at work. So some people will skip this section because they know far more about the e-world than it could possibly contain, and others will tiptoe through it with trepidation, wondering if any of it is likely to be even faintly comprehensible.

One thing is certain: e-awareness is an increasingly important part of the general awareness that underpins influence. While it may be possible to be influential without using electronic information or communication, it is very much more difficult. Email and websites are so widely used by policy makers, journals and professional organisations, and so much information is generated, stored and passed on by these methods, that not using them creates a real hurdle. It restricts available information, slows down access and response times, and, in the worst case, causes people to bypass you altogether in favour of people who can and do share these common tools of electronic communication. Whatever the reason for non-use of these tools – whether lack of training, restricted access at work, cost of computers or anything else – it is important to take action to resolve them, if you want to be effectively influential in today's world.

There are three main areas in which all health professionals need some e-awareness:

- how IT developments will contribute to the day-to-day running of mainstream health services
- what new services may develop based on electronic communication and developments
- how IT can contribute to personal professional development.

MIRROR MOMENT

What are your strengths and weaknesses regarding information technology? Use Table 12.1 to rate your current awareness. Which of your weaknesses worries you most, and why? This is the part to address as soon as possible.

TABLE 12.1 Essential IT awareness checklist

Skill	Know all about this	Can use it, need to develop	Not very sure	Not a clue
Using email				
Word processing				
Creating/reading spreadsheets				
Finding and searching specific websites				
General web searching				
Using bibliographic databases				
Creating graphs and charts				
Producing presentations				

IT and mainstream services

There is a major programme currently underway in the NHS to improve the use of information technology in support of clinical services. The National Programme for IT (NPfIT) is now being implemented by an agency known as 'Connecting for Health'. It involves a wide range of different elements from electronic booking of appointments to the transmission of images such as X-rays (*see* the 'need to know' information in Box 12.1). The use of email for communications between GPs and hospital consultants/departments, the electronic transmission of test results from laboratories to wards and/or GPs, and the online booking of out-patient appointments and investigations (called 'Choose and Book'), are already underway. Some areas have piloted other elements of the programme, such as the electronic patient record. Familiarity with the precise procedures for these activities can only be acquired once they are happening in your workplace, but experience of using computers and electronic communication in a variety of ways is an essential foundation for these additional uses. This has become all the more important because of the widespread use of information technology by patients and carers themselves, creating the expectation that they will be able to communicate with health professionals, obtain information and navigate the health system in the same way that they deal with on-line banking and shopping.

BOX 12.1 Need to know: NHS Connecting for Health

NHS Connecting for Health (CfH) is an agency of the Department of Health set up to deliver the National Programme for IT (NPfIT) in the NHS (www.connectingforhealth.nhs.uk).

This programme consists of seven key elements:

- *The NHS Care Records Service* (NHS CRS): providing 'an individual electronic NHS care record for every patient in England, securely accessible by patients and those caring for them'
- *Choose and Book*: an electronic appointment booking service 'offering patients greater choice of hospitals or clinics and more convenience in the date and time of their appointment'
- *The Electronic Prescription Service* (EPS): enabling prescriptions to be transferred from GP to pharmacy electronically
- *A new National Network* (N3): 'the IT infrastructure and broadband connectivity for the NHS so patient information can be shared between organisations'
- *'Contact'*: a central email and directory service for the NHS, to enable the secure transfer of patient information between staff
- *Picture Archiving and Communication Systems* (PACS): 'to capture, store, display and distribute static and moving digital medical images, providing clearer X-rays and scans and faster, more accurate diagnosis'
- *IT for GPs*, including the Quality Management and Analysis System (QMAS), support for the GPs' Quality and Outcomes Framework, and a system for GP to GP record transfer.

New services

NHS Direct and NHS Direct Online are examples of services that are built on electronic developments: in this case, the use of computer-based decision support algorithms combined with call-centre technology, and a website. Health channels on interactive digital television are another example of the way such technology will transform people's expectations of, and access to, health information and services.

PERSONAL DEVELOPMENT EXERCISE

Use a computer at work or at home, or an access terminal in a public place such as a pharmacy, to visit NHS Direct Online (www.nhsdirect.nhs.uk). Look at the material available on the website from the point of view of a lay person, and consider how easy it is to access, and how appropriate it might be for your patients, or your family and friends, to use. What are the pros and cons of providing health information in this way?

Other IT-dependent developments

In contrast to these 'on demand' services, there are several schemes in place that undertake routine follow-up of people with long-term conditions, or with complex medication routines, via the telephone.

There are also increasingly common examples of patients using technology to monitor their own condition at home, relaying results via the telephone to professionals elsewhere, and only being given advice or treatment when the results require it. Community matrons in some parts of the country are using these technologies as part of their case management role with patients, aimed at reducing the number of unplanned admissions to hospital.

IT and professional development

> *There are many ways of finding out information, and electronic libraries on line have revolutionised the ease of finding and retrieving information. Librarians are only too willing to help with setting up a search to review the literature.* (JULIA QUICKFALL)

The most obvious example of the potential for IT to contribute to professional development is the range of online learning resources available. These include online journals with searchable archives of articles and features, to entire post-registration courses delivered online. These have the major advantage of enabling people who would not be able to get time out of the workplace, or who are not currently working, to study, learn and gain knowledge and/or qualifications at a time and place that suits them.

Less formal uses of IT for development include looking up information on websites, downloading documents, exchanging questions and answers with network groups via email, and reading discussion boards.

So as well as the need to use technological developments coming into mainstream services, and to explain to patients entirely new IT-based services, all health and social care workers need IT skills to be able to take advantage of the relatively easy, cheap and comprehensive development opportunities on offer.

Key skills

The six indispensable skills in which you should be confident and competent in an increasingly IT-dependent health service are:

- *emailing*: to contact your network, exchange information, and send and receive documents. Your skill should extend to filing and 'house-keeping' your emails, and attaching your automatic electronic 'signature'
- *internet searching*: to find information about key people and organisations, and relevant publications, or find out about patients' experiences
- *database searching*: both online research databases, to find articles and books on a particular subject, or evidence to support practice, and 'good practice'

databases, to find out who else is doing innovative work in your field
- *website navigation*: of organisations such as statutory and regulatory bodies, government departments, charities and lobby groups, to find specific information, or people to contact. It is useful to have developed your list of 'favourites' so that you can quickly visit relevant websites
- *word processing*: most documents involved in influencing work (policy statements, consultations, guidance, publications and journal articles) are created, edited, shared, read and amended in their word-processed forms. Handwritten documents, or comments on documents, are too slow and labour-intensive, and fewer and fewer people have the administrative support to work in this way. Word-processing skills should include using 'track changes' to provide alternative text for a document
- *presentations*: using computer software to prepare and present visual presentations is now so common that other methods of presentation tend to look amateurish and diminish the credibility of the speaker – except in special circumstances. It is worth having the ability to put together a presentation in this way, and essential to know how to deliver such a presentation.

These skills open up access to huge amounts of information, and enable you to build a network of contacts and exert your influence, much more quickly and effectively than other methods. There will always be a place for letters (*see* Chapter 23) and for the telephone: but they must now be used in conjunction with electronic methods of communication and information gathering.

Acquiring the skills

> *Do not feel that you should be able to do these things without support and do not be afraid to ask for help.* (Christine Singleton)

Many health and social care workers will have and use some of the skills discussed above regularly, if not daily, in their work or at home. But if you don't already have the specific computer skills discussed above, how can you acquire them? Such is the importance of these skills in all walks of life that there are many national and local initiatives in place to teach and build on the basics:
- public libraries run courses, often without charge, to teach people how to access the internet, and carry out basic web searching
- schools and colleges hold evening classes in computer skills at levels from basic to advanced, often at subsidised costs
- universities provide computer skills modules to support a range of courses, on the basis that computer use is essential to manage assignments
- medical or nursing library staff may offer formal or informal training in literature searching and conducting web searches
- most employers have software manuals that can be used to develop specific skills such as using databases or spreadsheets

- some organisations provide 'at desk' training, or internal courses, run by the IT department, to teach people how to use the network system specific to the organisation
- manufacturers installing new computer systems often offer free training for staff as part of the package.

Finally, of course, there are the most informal routes to gaining these skills: asking other people to show you. Children are often the most useful, but administrative staff at work may also be able to help, if you are prepared to learn in small doses when you and they can snatch some time.

> *If information processing is not your job but is necessary for you to carry out your job effectively, then get to know your IT department personnel and do not hesitate to contact them.* (CHRISTINE SINGLETON)

Whatever opportunities you find, it is essential to take advantage of them. Start from the premise that you are not going to have to pay for this training – but be prepared to do so if necessary. Not only is it a huge investment in developing your awareness, but when you come to exert your influence – on your trust, professional association, peers or government – it will be quicker, easier and more effective if you can use email, word processing and information from the web.

CHECKLIST FOR ACTION

Have you:

- visited the NHS Direct website (www.nhsdirect.nhs.uk)?
- identified any gaps in your IT skills?
- found an opportunity to fill those gaps through a course or help from someone who is competent in the relevant skills?

CHAPTER 13

Being aware of policy

> *Three top tips on being aware of policy: identify the key drivers of those you want to influence; understand the national policy context; and articulate the local picture.* (SUZANNE HILTON)

It is hard to avoid thinking about government policy when you work in health and social care. It is a very political arena, with politicians from all parties keen to be associated with the successes of the NHS and good social care, and to be heard on all the key issues. They tend to be equally keen to make statements, implement change and re-structure organisations whenever something goes wrong, or simply to stamp their mark on the services after an election. The media reports all the speeches and activity, and policy initiatives are passed down to service level to be implemented, measured and reported on.

So most workers in health and social care have experienced new initiatives, pilot projects, organisational mergers, changing lines of accountability, performance management, and the collision of professional and policy priorities. So, do you know all about government health and social care policy?

MIRROR MOMENT

Think about what you know about the current government's health or social care policies. Can you describe one policy in a few sentences, and say what the government's rationale for it is? Where do you get this information from – and how hard to do you look for it? Maybe it is what is reported in your weekly journal, or what your manager tells you is happening. If you had to give a presentation to colleagues about it next week, where would you go for the full story?

What do we mean by 'policy'?

'Policy' is made visible by all the different decisions taken by the government of the day about healthcare and social care. Those decisions cover the financing and organisation of health and social care, the workforce that delivers it, the nature and scope of services, commissioning and procurement, involvement of service users, training and education of staff, research and development programmes, ethical issues . . . and so on. Ideally, the raft of decisions, made at different times by different ministers, reflects an over-arching plan: often contained in a major policy document such as a White Paper or National Service Framework. So the many individual 'policies' are like the little bones on a fish bone, connected to the big structural bone of policy direction, and enabling the whole thing to move forwards. As an example, the recent human resources policy for the NHS used the heading 'More staff, working differently'. This was the overall policy statement, with the direction set in a major document called *HR in the NHS*. Contributing to the delivery of this policy were a wide range of smaller-scale policies, including initiatives on recruitment and retention, improving working lives, changing professional roles, updating professional regulation, introducing new practitioners, and so on.

Developing awareness of policy

> *Be clear about what the policies actually say as often what is described as a 'must-do' is actually advisory only.* (Judith Ellis)

Many people have a superficial awareness of some of the government policies that affect their area of work. They pick up an outline of what is happening from articles in newspapers or their professional journals, by listening to discussion in the workplace, reading in-house summaries provided by employers and managers, or looking at web-based discussion boards. These are useful methods to alert you that something is happening that will affect your organisation or area of work. The danger is that you pick up incomplete or inaccurate information, or mistake rumour or local interpretation for the full story. This is not enough to enable you to influence policy – and it is a mistake to rattle off a letter or email with your opinion and suggestions, on the basis of such information. You are likely to be ignored, your reputation could be damaged, and you will be embarrassed.

Working in the Department of Health, I regularly received correspondence from health professionals suggesting change or commenting on policies that demonstrated with painful clarity that they had not kept up with developments, or had not taken the trouble to understand them. Worse, some of these letters came via ministers' offices, because the practitioner had written directly to the minister. The impression it left of the people working in the service – who genuinely wanted to make things better for patients and for the service as a whole – was undoubtedly a poor one, and did not inspire confidence. These were not the people who were invited to sit on advisory groups, comment on documents or attend policy workshops.

> *Keep right up to date with national and local strategic priorities and be ready to use them when appropriate.* (Sandra Mellors)

Taking the time to make yourself fully aware of a policy area will pay dividends.

It will ensure you give a good impression as you attempt to influence the future direction or implementation of policy, by helping you contribute constructively to the debate. The impact of your contribution and your professional standing with influential people will be enhanced. To improve services for patients or clients, or simply to get yourself noticed in the corridors of power – or something in between – you need to have more than a superficial awareness of health policy.

Building policy awareness

> *Keep up to date: read summaries and only the whole document if you need to, so you have a broad knowledge about all things and can do what you are asked – you can always go into more depth when needed.* (JUDITH WHITTAM)

Policy on health and social care is a huge field. Unless you have a particularly challenging assignment for a higher degree, you probably don't need to study the health and social care policies of the current government in their entirety. Instead, identify the area where you want to influence, and focus on that. It may be:

- your specialist clinical area (such as cancer chemotherapy, residential care, or abnormal pregnancy)
- the service you provide or work in (adoption, counselling, community pharmacy)
- an area you want to become an 'expert' in (*see* Chapter 15 about the use of the term 'expert') such as joint commissioning or social care funding
- something that affects you personally (such as informal carers or infertility)
- something you feel strongly about (such as residential home closures or the career path for healthcare scientists).

Although you will need to focus on the area you have chosen, it is still important to know something of the wider context, as background against which to set all the things you learn about the specific subject. Often this is contained in one document: the 'big picture' plan. It is impossible for this book to point to a particular document, because they change in a relatively short time. But it is probably one you have heard of by reading journals, and is likely to have been 'launched' with some fanfare.

PERSONAL DEVELOPMENT EXERCISE

Look for the latest document published by the Department of Health (in whichever country of the UK you work) that gives an overview of the issues facing health and social care, and which contains plans for 5–10 years ahead. Pick out the main themes, and the key issues that the document says are important to (a) retain and (b) change. This provides the background for policies related to the area you are interested in, and about to focus on.

Zooming in

With this overview of the general direction of policy as the backbone, you can now explore your particular 'bone'. Four steps should make you very much better informed:

- look at relevant websites on your subject
- read *full* policy documents or statements on it
- check for linked *local* documents and policies
- review your informal sources, such as journal articles and opinions.

Websites

Start with the relevant government departments. Each of the UK countries has its own health department, which combines responsibility for health and social care. Other government departments may have equally relevant material because of their intersecting responsibilities: those handling education, crime and social disorder, housing and social inclusion, business and entrepreneurialism, and welfare and benefits will all be relevant. There is a wealth of policy information very easily accessible from these sites. With a bit of experimental searching (it is easier on each occasion) you should be able to find:

- all policy documents, statements and guidance documents related to your subject: these are the foundation stones of the policy, and you should bookmark them, print them off or send for full copies of the most recent ones, as they are essential reference sources
- names of ministers and senior officials in the department and their individual areas of responsibility
- texts of ministerial speeches on the subject (*see* 'need to know' information in Box 13.1) – these will often set out the 'vision' for the policy area
- related documents and information – find these by following the links suggested on the site you have accessed or to other sites; or by scrolling down to find earlier documents on the subject that have now been superseded. It is worth thinking laterally about other places to look for related documents that may not have a built-in link: for example, check the R&D pages to see what research has been, or is currently being, funded on the subject by the department. *See* Box 13.2 for an example of the information found on the subject of domestic violence, starting from a search of the Department of Health website
- the name of the policy lead, or other people working on policy in the field you are interested in. If not explicitly stated, you may find it on the inside of policy documents under 'author' or 'for further information, contact . . .', or in a consultation document (*see* below). Even if this person is an administrative contact for additional copies, they can provide the name of the policy people involved
- consultation documents: these can provide an enormous amount of useful information. Often a consultation document will rehearse the history of a piece of work or a set of policies; explain the issues that necessitate change; set out a number of options that are being considered; and list the organisations that are being consulted, so providing a ready-made list of key stakeholders in the field.

The options are particularly interesting, as, once the consultation is over and the policy decision made, they are a record of routes that the government decided *not* to go down – and you might want to explore the reasons why. If the consultation is still open, you might want to respond, as an individual or by consulting a group you belong to (*see* Chapter 20). Responses to consultations are also usually posted on the website alongside the closed consultations, so you can see what stance various organisations and individuals took to the proposals, how much support there was for each option, and so on

- communications about the policy: you will be able to find the press releases that accompany ministerial announcements, and sometimes sets of slides from talks given on the topic by senior policy makers
- downloadable resources: either from the main government site, or linked sites, these may include 'fact-files', information sheets, presentations from conferences, algorithms etc.

BOX 13.1 Need to know: ministerial speeches

Speeches are usually written for ministers by civil servants, then reviewed and redrafted in line with the minister's comments. Special advisors to ministers may also have an input. However, ministers will also amend the speech at the last minute to reflect their latest thinking, new information or feedback. Speeches often contain one or more announcements relating to the subject – for example, announcing a change in policy, a new initiative to be introduced, or new funding. To be sure that these are picked up, they are usually introduced specifically with phrases like: 'Today I can announce that . . .'. So ministerial speeches are a good place to check that the rumour you heard about '£5 million for research into . . .' or 'the threshold for self-funding of care to be raised' is correct.

As there can be major changes to a speech in the hours before it is given, and even while on the platform, you need to be sure that the speech you are reading is accurate. Note that a speech marked 'Checked against delivery' means that it records what the minister actually said on the day, not what was in the original script of the speech.

BOX 13.2 Information on domestic violence from the Department of Health website

The search term 'domestic violence' on the Department of Health website led to:

- reports of conferences on domestic abuse
- a resource handbook for professionals
- results of surveys on domestic abuse
- a telephone helpline
- ministerial speeches on the subject
- a downloadable audit tool
- policy documents
- relevant legislation
- nationally collated statistics.

It is worth checking when documents were published, and when areas of the site were last updated – sometimes you will find pages that have not been updated for some months. See this as an opportunity to contact the department to ask for an update.

Also bear in mind the Freedom of Information Act requirement for public bodies to provide you with information you ask for on a particular subject: if you are looking for something in particular, or feel that you don't have the full picture, you can request information from a government department, local authority, NHS organisation, or any other public body. However, it is no-one's interest for public sector workers to spend large amounts of time and photocopying budgets responding to unnecessary, speculative or trivial requests, so two essential 'first steps' before you contemplate such a request are:

- making sure the information isn't already accessible through the website, papers (such as published meeting papers) or publications. It is amazing how much information is already available, particularly through minutes of meetings
- being sure that you really need it: you are not asking just as an exercise to test the system, or because you have a passing interest, but because you need the information for a specific purpose. *See* Box 13.3 for more on using the Freedom of Information Act.

BOX 13.3 Using the Freedom of Information Act

The Freedom of Information Act 2000 enables people to access information held by public authorities in two ways:

- *through publication schemes*: these make some information available to the public as a matter of routine, without a specific request being required
- *through a general right of access*: public authorities must respond to requests for information within 20 working days. This right came into force on 1 January 2005.

There are some exemptions to the information that must be provided by public authorities (such as NHS organisations, local authorities and government departments). These include, amongst others:

- information related to policy formulation, ministerial communications, law officers' advice (i.e. the legal advice given to ministers) and the operation of ministerial private offices
- information 'for the effective conduct of public affairs'
- information reasonably accessible to the applicant by other means.

Each of these exemptions is subject to its own guidance. See the website of the Information Commissioner's Office www.ico.gov.uk for full details.

Reading the full document

Very few people read full policy documents. Of course you can see why when you try – they can be lengthy, full of jargon and acronyms, and tediously detailed on the subject of past policy successes, while light on practical information about the future.

But the better documents are tightly written descriptions of key steps to be taken, set in a helpful summary context, and demonstrating how the next pieces of the policy jigsaw fit into the 'big picture'. And being one of the people who has read the whole thing, and understands how it fits together, what is going to happen next, and what the intended outcome is, gives you an enormous amount of authority when you come to contribute, formally or informally. The approach I find works best is:

- print off the whole thing so that you can refer backwards and forwards more easily than you can on a screen
- read it through once from start to finish without stopping for notes – it is surprising how much you will retain and be able to recall at a key moment
- read it through again with a highlighter pen to hand, and mark the key bullet points, paragraphs or summaries
- write any notes, comments or questions on the document itself, as a separate piece of paper has a habit of separating itself and wasting all the work you have done
- if the paper is thick and unwieldy, you might want to make your own one-page crib sheet that is more easily taken with you to meetings, pinned up on a notice board, or used to brief colleagues in a team meeting. Use bullet points to remind you of key facts: what is going to happen, the key numbers and figures, and the timescale.

Finding linked local documents

When you have finished this initial reading, follow up leads such as references to previous policy documents or related pieces of work. Then you can ask around, and look around, in your own organisation (website, board papers, team meetings) to see what impact the national policy has had on local action, what frontline staff's reactions to it has been, and who is leading on it in your organisation. If you have made yourself aware of policy in this way, and you are keen to influence policy, then your local lead on the topic should be part of your network of contacts (*see* Chapter 14 on networks). Understanding the national policy picture and direction will make these local documents and actions meaningful – that is why it is most useful to do your research in this order.

Reviewing informal sources

Now that you have the real, national picture on policies related to your area of interest, and have looked at the local response and implementation, it is useful to return to those more informal sources of information that, taken alone, gave the more superficial view. Articles in journals, statements from interest groups, professional organisations and unions, newspaper articles and opinion pieces from commentators can be very useful at this stage. They provide different perspectives on the policy, they give alternative, conflicting and sometimes opposite views of what it all means, and they highlight possible alternative courses of action. Importantly, they may set out what they think the consequences of the policy direction may be. Remember that they may or may not be right: but it is useful to know what concerns there are, and how sensitive or difficult, supported or opposed, the proposals or policy are likely to be.

To get the most value from this informal source of thinking on the subject, get as wide a range of responses as possible. Read a range of journals, looking at articles, editorials, opinion pieces and the letters page. Look for responses or statements from research centres and 'think-tanks', unions and patients' groups, as well as your own professional organisation. Listen to frontline staff as they discuss the topic, and read papers from, or attend, board meetings to see what the directors are saying. Ask the patients' forum, a support group or a charity in the field how they see things.

This is not a one-off activity – your awareness of a particular area needs to be kept up to date by continuous exposure to information from all the sources outlined above. The good news is that it quickly becomes second nature to acquire this information, to read policy documents, find the key points and spot the trends. The language and processes quickly become familiar (*see* Chapter 25 for more on the policy process), as will the names of ministers, civil servants, clinical leads, researchers and commentators in the field. Suddenly you will feel like, and sound like, an expert in the area – and your potential to influence policy will be enormous.

Practical aspects of developing policy awareness

Make the collection of information easier for yourself by automating it whenever possible. Sign up to have electronic newsletters, and news briefings, delivered to your computer desktop: you may need to make this your home computer to ensure you can see them quickly and regularly. Also – or instead, if you really don't have access to a computer – make sure you are on the circulation list for updates, newsletters and other information sent out by relevant organisations. Professional organisations and unions will do this as part of your membership.

Add relevant government departments' press release, policy statement and publication lists to your list of favourites in your search engine. It is much easier to check regularly with one click of the mouse than by entering the website address and starting at the home page every time.

It is a good idea to start a file for each subject you are investigating, to keep policy documents, copies of articles, meeting papers and other material together. As you prepare for meetings, or write articles or letters yourself, it will be much easier if you can find the titles of documents, references, facts and figures you need in one place.

Having done all this work to become an expert on the policy developments in your area of interest, you may want to use it for other things. Consider writing an article about it, or using it as the basis for an assignment if you are doing a university course. You could offer to arrange a local study day, or a presentation to a meeting on the subject. All these raise your profile, help you think through the implications of the policy, and prepare you for action to influence change.

PORTFOLIO POINTER

Put a note in your professional portfolio to record the fact that you have prepared a file on a particular policy area (include the crib sheet you produced), and record any other activities you undertake as a result, such as briefing a meeting or writing an article.

PERSONAL DEVELOPMENT EXERCISE

Decide on an area and explore policy on that area as described in this section. Visit websites of relevant government departments and find out the minister responsible for the area, and the official leading work on it. Produce the one-page crib sheet on the main points of the latest policy developments, and put a copy in your portfolio. Then contact the local lead for this policy area in your organisation and let them know that you are interested. Ask if you can shadow them for a day, or have a meeting with them to find out more about local plans.

CHECKLIST FOR ACTION

Check that you have:

- put a copy of the policy 'crib sheet' you produced in your portfolio
- 'bookmarked' key websites on your computer
- contacted a local leader to let them know you are interested in this area.

CHAPTER 14

Creating, using and maintaining 'networks'

Networking is a bit like keeping friendships, it takes time and effort and nurturing. (JOANNA PARKER)

'Networking' is such an abused and over-used term, you could be forgiven for thinking there is no point in discussing it here. It has become a catch-all phrase for any time spent with other people that isn't a formal meeting or conference session, even if you spend it complaining about the lateness of the trains or the quality of the coffee. As with 'brainstorming' and 'thinking outside the box', we need a new respectable phrase to restore the reputation of what is actually a very powerful and useful activity.

Networking, done well, is the essential connection between awareness and influence. Sharing information, advice, support, contacts and learning with a wide range of other people builds your own awareness far faster than you could ever manage alone. And knowing people to talk to, write to, consult, bring in to a project and put forward for a job gives you many more avenues for influence than you could possibly access in isolation. The active processes connecting these two involve effort, trust, integrity, continuity and openness. These are what keep networks humming, growing and strengthening. They are also what distinguish networking from a mere series of disconnected conversations.

MIRROR MOMENT

Do you consider yourself to have a network? If so, think about what makes these people, and your relationship with them, different from others you may have worked with, spoken to or met in the past. How active have you been in contacting these people, and how do you do it?

Practical networking

There are many books available that look at the sociological and anthropological theories of networking. This isn't one of them. This chapter looks at networks from a purely practical perspective, suggesting ways in which you can build up your networks as part of your project to be more influential in the health services.

Why network?

> *Other people and their experiences are potentially your biggest asset, so time spent building networks generally pays off, as does sharing work and ideas.* (Deb Lapthorne)

There are two kinds of answer to this: the selfish ones and the altruistic ones. For most people, the motivation for networking is a healthy mix of both. If someone has entirely selfish motives, their contacts will soon realise this, and their network will tend to weaken and break down. If someone's motives are entirely altruistic – they are either very odd, or lying.

Selfish reasons for building a network are:

- to increase your career opportunities
- to build up your knowledge base
- to try to meet 'important' people
- to stop your job becoming boring
- to make a name for yourself
- to help you get your next job.

Altruistic motives are:

- to help others in their careers
- to contribute to other people's personal development
- to enhance your professional skills
- to improve services for patients
- to help make better health policies
- to 'give something back' to the profession.

> *These are not mystical or always useful. Build alliances with colleagues, take time to help them, and in due course they will help you.* (Judy Hargadon)

In the context of this book, the motivation for building networks is a nice mix of the two: it is to broaden your awareness of what is going on in the health services and the professions, in order to influence change for the better. Along the way, this is also very likely to help you get your next job or professional opportunity, and to help improve services. Lots of wins all round – if it is done well.

> *Interest begets interest. If you are sufficiently interested in someone's area then hopefully they will reciprocate when you are trying to engage support. This is not sycophancy or manipulation but a way of engaging with people. It is a way of 'banking' information and knowledge about people who may be able to help you in the future.* (Maureen Williams)

PERSONAL DEVELOPMENT EXERCISE

Try listing the people you consider to be in your network at the moment. Exclude people in your immediate workplace or team, and list only those whom you don't have day-to-day contact with, under functional headings such as those shown in Figure 14.1. Look at which areas you have most and least contacts in. Which would you like to build up – and why?

People from relevant voluntary groups and charities
People in similar areas of practice
Educators and researchers in the field
You
People involved in national policy on the subject
People in your professional organisation
Journal contracts

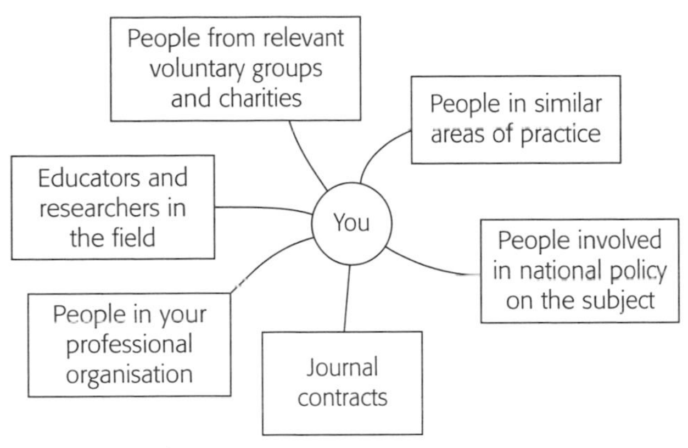

Figure 14.1 Mapping your network

Who do you want in your network?

It is important to engage more widely than your own organisation and your own occupational group – you must network outside your comfort zone. (ALISON NORMAN)

There is no right answer to who 'should' be in your network. It will depend on what your plans and ambitions are. If you want to develop a career in research eventually, clearly you would want to make new contacts in education and research groups. But you might also want to connect with leaders and innovators in the clinical field that you are interested in; with policy makers who decide how research programmes are commissioned; and with charities that fund research projects or provide travel bursaries. If you want to change the way a particular client group is perceived, treated or involved in services, you will want to build on your network of organisational contacts, special interest group leaders, media people and lobbyists. The aim should be to have a network diagram with lots of boxes of various sizes, rather than a few bigger, neater boxes – think of a bunch of mixed flowers rather than a couple of perfect carnations! Figure 14.2 shows an example of a network and a 'wish list' of new contacts to go with it.

While it is important to build a network through positive action to find these specific people that you have identified, it is just as valuable to nurture the unexpected,

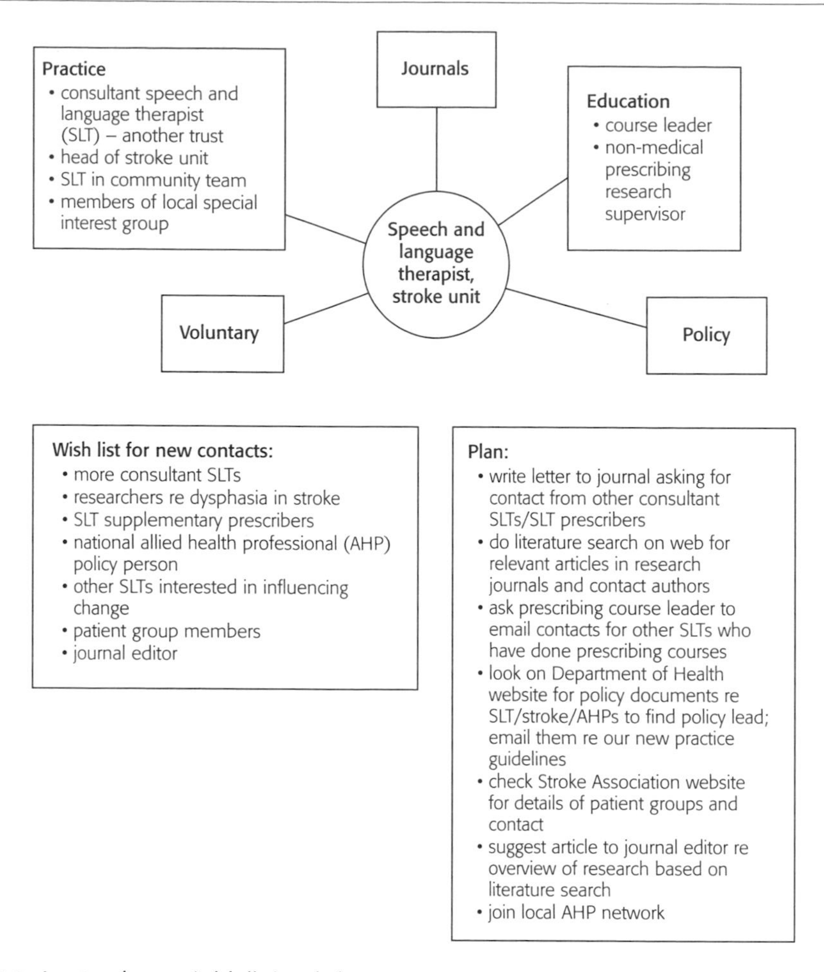

Figure 14.2 A network map, 'wish list' and plan

chance contact. There are opportunities everywhere to link up with people you could not have planned to meet: such as the person sitting next to you at a conference, or someone you start a conversation with on a train. It is surprising how often these contacts come into their own many years after they were first made, providing they were sufficiently nurtured to take root in the early days.

> *One of the commonest mistakes people make is to be 'invisible' and hard to contact. Always have a stock of business cards with you and follow up a meeting or conversation with an email or phone call if it has been particularly beneficial.* (Sue Norman)

It is important to bear in mind that network contacts are not necessarily friends. Some will become so; some may become mentors. Others will remain simply part of your network: but, if you have maintained your network with honesty, integrity and the requisite degree of effort, there will be a warmth in these contacts that makes it easy to pick up again after a gap, and disposes both of you to make and respond to requests when the time comes.

PORTFOLIO POINTER

Put your current network map, and your notes on how you would like to build it up, into your professional portfolio. Then you can look back at it in a year's time, and see how successful you have been in building up your contacts.

Growing your network

> *Networks are essential – but it is a two-way process, don't just use your colleagues in the network. Feedback how the information is used and publicly recognise ideas that came from others.* (Barbara Stuttle)

When you know what sort of contacts you are aiming to make, there are many ways to go about it. For example:

- *responding to a journal article*: if you see an article on your subject by someone you don't know, write to them to express interest, or comment on what they say. You could offer to send information on your own work, or your organisation's protocols, or, if what they have written about is sufficiently novel or challenging, ask to visit their site. The author's email address may be included with their details alongside the articles. If not, the organisation they work for will usually be mentioned, and can be found via its website for an email address. If all else fails, you can write to the journal and ask them to forward your letter/email to the author (an example of the effort you may need to put in to build your network – don't give up at the first hurdle). It is possible that you won't get a reply – in which case, do follow up politely after a few weeks, in case your original email or letter got lost – but it often works. People generally do like to share what they know and what they're doing, and to learn from others
- *talking to a conference speaker*: there is always that moment when a conference session ends and the delegates stampede for the doors as if they haven't already had three cups of coffee and several Danish pastries since arriving at the venue. But you might also notice two or three people fighting against the tide to get to the front of the hall to have a word with the speakers as they leave the stage, podium or front row. This is the place to be. If you are at the conference, the topics should be of some relevance to you. The speakers have been selected for their input on these topics. Whether you agree or disagree with what they have said, or could have done it better yourself, this is an opportunity to speak face-to-face with them. It is always worth picking up a point with them, asking a question or at least asking if you can contact them later to discuss their experience, knowledge, project or whatever they were speaking about. Most speakers are well aware that they don't have all the answers, and they are not doing anything exceptional. They are

usually glad to know about others' work in the same area, and to swap resources or ideas. When the speakers are from national organisations, or *do* appear to have a lot of the answers, this is an opportunity to put yourself on their radar as someone interested in, or working in, the same field. Where else could you walk up and introduce yourself to the head of a professional organisation, a Department of Health policy lead, or a national clinical director? They may be in a hurry and surrounded by others, and you may have to wait five minutes – but you can give them your name and what you do, and a few complimentary words about their presentation or speech, and say you'll email them after the conference, in less than a minute. Follow-up effectively, and you may have a rewarding new contact

- *one word of warning*: if the speaker is a real VIP of any kind, you may not get near them. Don't force it: you don't want to appear aggressive. You can still email later and say 'I heard your presentation at such and such an event and . . .'
- *writing to a journal*: *see* Chapter 23 for more on this. You can write in response to someone else's letter, starting a dialogue that can continue outside the pages of the journal if you give your email address. Or you can write to ask people with a specific interest or experience to contact you, and build up your contacts from those who respond. It is useful to write to journals other than those you read regularly, and to those aimed at other health professions than your own. This is a good way to build up cross-professional networks
- *joining a special interest group or relevant professional organisation*: many professionals join their organisation or union solely for its indemnity insurance or employment services. Valuable as these are, there is usually much more to these organisations than this, including groups or forums for special interests. Joining one of these is essential to network building. By definition, the people in them want to network with others, and they share a common interest and area of practice. This is a shortcut to finding numerous useful contacts in one easy step. Not all of the forum members will be equally active, or equally relevant to the purpose for which you are networking. But no contact is ever wasted, and even those who stay on the periphery of your network may one day develop a new importance. Bear in mind that you don't need to confine yourself to one special interest group: if you are a speech and language therapist (SLT) in the community for example, you might belong to one group that shares your special interest in autistic spectrum disorders and language; another connecting SLTs who offer clinical supervision to peers; and a local forum looking at services to a particular estate. All these will usefully widen your personal network of contacts, and all will benefit from what you can offer other members
- *looking for shadowing opportunities*: sometimes these are specifically advertised, which makes it easier – all you have to do is negotiate the time to do it as part of your personal development. But if there are no opportunities that excite you on offer, there is no reason why you cannot identify someone you think would be useful in your network, and ask them for the chance to spend a day with them. By treating the day professionally, and continuing contact appropriately afterwards, you can begin to build the networking relationship. Do make sure that you have

a reason for asking that particular person, however, and a clear idea of what you want from the shadowing experience. Unfortunately, people sometimes write to very senior and busy people in vague but optimistic terms about how much they would enjoy shadowing them 'for my personal development'. You are much more likely to get a positive response to your request if you:

- list some specific objectives for the day
- say how you will prepare for the day (what you will read, whose advice you will seek locally, how you will research their organisation)
- suggest some benefits for the person you will shadow – information you could share, documents you could bring, a visit you could arrange
- recognise that you might not spend all day with the key individual, but would value the chance to spend time with others in their organisation too

If such a day should be arranged, there are three cardinal rules: don't cancel it; write or email afterwards with thanks and to say how it benefited you; and follow up the contacts you make on the day promptly afterwards

- *reading a different journal*: this is a good way to get a completely new perspective on your subject, and to identify new contacts. It is easy to get into the habit of reading one journal, knowing who writes for them, what the editorial view is, and who sends letters in. Another journal in your own profession, or, better, one read by another profession, is completely different. You can find out what GPs really think of nurses who operate, why pharmacists are concerned about a new contract, and how social care workers feel about working in teams with nurses, by reading their journals. At the same time, it becomes easier to spot those issues that connect healthcare workers, and to think more broadly about service matters. Building up contacts from outside one's own profession should always be on a networker's 'to do' list
- *doing a site visit*: the difference between seeing a project or person *in situ*, and exchanging emails or reading articles about them, is vast. On a site visit you will meet more people unexpectedly, see the reality that may not be apparent in the written version, and have a chance to make more of an impression on more people. Of course it isn't easy to take yourself off on lots of visits, so they need to be worthwhile. Expect to exchange emails, papers and phone calls before you arrange a visit: you need to save your time and your manager's benediction for something really worthwhile. Like shadowing, put the work in beforehand, be clear about what you want to get out of the visit, and follow up afterwards. Also, in both site visits and shadowing, remember the impression you make on everybody you meet, not just the 'main man' you have come to see
- *holding a meeting or open day*: why not invite people to come to you? By taking charge of the process, you can be sure that you have a good chance of meeting some new people with an interest in your field or cause, whom you can subsequently contact again. Of course this takes more time and effort than other ways of finding new contacts, and doing it badly can be worse than not doing it at all. So only attempt it if you have the time and support. If you don't, then use other people's events to the maximum, and let them handle the hassle!

- *using other meetings*: it is fashionable to complain that meetings are a waste of time, and joke that they 'an alternative to work'. If they are wasting your time, then either you shouldn't be there, or you are not using them properly (*see* Chapter 19). One of the ways of using them is to enlarge your network. So, before and after the official business of the meeting, instead of scanning the papers you should already have read, looking out of the window or phoning home:
  - introduce yourself to anyone in the room you don't know, and find out who they are, where they are from and what their role in the meeting is (some of this you can crib from the list of names on the previous minutes, then impress them because when they say 'I'm Andy Jones from A&E' you can say 'Oh yes, you're the emergency nurse practitioner, aren't you?')
  - actively look for connections between your work or interest and theirs ('Can I talk to you sometime about triage protocols?')
  - note names and numbers or email addresses directly into your diary or organiser – if you jot them on the agenda they are likely to get lost
  - talk to the people you already know, to cement relations
  - introduce people who don't know each other – this helps build their networks, and establishes you as someone who knows people
- During the meeting, for maximum effect, make sure you introduce yourself clearly when invited to do so. Look round as you speak, smile and meet people's eyes, so that they are more likely to remember you, and take the chance to say what you do and where you are from, and, if you have the chance, why you have an interest in the issue of the meeting. Many times at meetings, when 'going round the table', people either appear pathologically shy (incapable of saying their own name, unable to meet anyone's eye, and unsure of their right to be present); or unspeakably arrogant (saying their name only in a throw-away manner that suggests everyone else round the table should instantly recognise it, and know their awesome reputation). This is a chance to make an impression on people, and it is important to do it with confidence.

Don't be precious about sharing ideas and information. (Kay East)

MIRROR MOMENT

How easy do you find it to talk to people you don't know in a meeting room? Is this routine for you, or a vision of hell? If you're not comfortable with introducing yourself and speaking up in this way, it might help to write down what you will say beforehand, so that you have the reassurance of notes – though you should rehearse enough not to need to look at them constantly. Then it is a question of practice: use every meeting or group you go to, to drill yourself to look round, smile, and speak clearly. It might help to notice how poor other people – even senior people – can be at this. It is quite likely that people will end up copying you because they see you as the one with the confidence, whatever you feel internally!

Maintaining a network

Make an effort – send notes, cards of congratulations, sympathy etc. Always try to write to anyone who receives a gong or promotion. (Monica Fletcher)

Suppose, by using the sort of opportunities described above, that you have enlarged your network to include a wide variety of people, from various professions and related organisations, who share your interests. How can you keep this network going, building the trust and relationships that will keep it active and engaged? Some straightforward practical points are:

- note down full contact details as soon as possible after making the contact, in a relatively permanent form like a notebook or personal organiser (paper or palm-top). A diary is no good if you have to copy everything out laboriously into the new one at the end of every year. But back up electronic records, and decide how you will retrieve your contacts if you lose the book!
- also note down something about why you are in touch with the person. Just keeping their business card won't help you remember whether they are the person who is piloting a new kind of coronary care unit (CCU) outreach service, or introducing hypnotherapy sedation, when you look at it again in six months' time
- make a follow-up contact soon after the first, if only to say 'it was good to see you at the conference' or 'thanks for giving me your email address'. This makes the other person realise that you were (and are) serious about sharing information, not just passing the time in a dull meeting
- respond quickly to contacts or requests for information from others in your network – don't let them languish for weeks in your inbox. If you can't help, reply to say so, and if possible suggest somewhere else to go for the information
- take the trouble to help: it is always tempting when you are busy to reply quickly that you can't help, rather than searching out a copy of an article or phoning up another contact for information. But you will want people to do it for you, so invest in gaining goodwill in your network
- take the time to be warm in your response. It doesn't take much longer to say or type 'hope to see you at the conference next month' or 'hope this is useful', and a curt-sounding message can damage relations as much as a warm one can build. No-one wants to feel that they are being addressed like an irritating child
- remember that 'give and take' is the essence of a network. Sometimes you will seem to be giving all the time – but it will even up over time, if you are using your network properly
- the way you conduct yourself in 'public' – and a network is a very public, if largely virtual, place – is important. The NHS may be the second largest employer in

Europe, but it is also a surprisingly small world, and the more specialist your role, the truer that is. People have long memories, and they talk to each other, and meet up at events. Lots of NHS people have NHS people as partners! Word gets around, and you simply never know when you will cross paths with someone who has heard of you through third parties involved in your network. I could give many examples, both positive and negative, of how this web of reputation has worked

- aim to make sure that people only hear good things about you – after all, it is very much in your interests!

> *Network with the right people – information sources, power brokers etc. Give out your details freely. Keep a note of contacts and use them.* (Fran Woodard)

PERSONAL DEVELOPMENT EXERCISE

Pick two or three of the actions listed above under 'Growing your network', and put them into practice over the next few weeks. Aim to add another four people to your network. As well as deliberately seeking out new people, remember to be alert to chance encounters that may be just as fruitful.

CHECKLIST FOR ACTION

Have you:

- mapped your current network?
- identified the gaps where you want to find new contacts?
- found four more people to fill those gaps?

SECTION 3

Developing influence

CHAPTER 15

How to become an expert

Be passionate about something you know you need to be passionate about and don't be ashamed of it. Write about it, get published, even just a letter to a professional journal. (JOANNA PARKER)

Surely the way to become an expert is to qualify, study, practise, publish, teach and research over a period of years? You can't just 'become' an expert by following a few tips, can you?

In the proper sense of the word expert, the answer would be 'no'. But in the sense of an expert as someone who is informed in their field, a known name, readily associated with a particular topic, and called upon to comment, publish, teach and speak at conferences, then you can become one in very short order. Becoming an 'informal expert' is not difficult, because relatively few people bother to put in the extra effort and commitment required.

For those who do, the effort is quickly repaid and a virtuous 'expert circle' develops: you write a few articles about something, people invite you to speak at study days on the strength of them, you learn more about the subject in preparing to speak about it, and become more knowledgeable. Then you write some more, and people think you're an expert on the subject, so they invite you to speak more and you study more and become more expert . . . By now, your name is your badge: it is recognisable, and associated in people's minds with 'your' topic. It is an excellent way of becoming influential, providing you with the platforms, the audience and the authority to argue your case.

PERSONAL DEVELOPMENT EXERCISE

Look at the journal you read most often, over a period of a couple of months, and note the names of authors of articles, columnists and letter writers. Are there familiar ones? Whom do you associate with, for example, writing on prescribing, elder abuse, or continence care? You will find that the same names come up repeatedly. You can test this by putting a subject into a search on one of the online archives: in a list of articles on your topic, there will always be names that crop up several times.

The 'expert'

Does this mean that these people are charlatans, conning the readership by recycling themselves endlessly? Not if they are regularly improving their knowledge of the subject, in order to provide something useful every time. And that is the key. You do have to know what you are talking about, and keep up to date on your topic. This is not difficult, and quickly becomes part of your professional life. But as many people do not make the time to do it, it is actually quite easy to be one paper, one article or one study ahead of the crowd – and to use that as the basis for your expertise.

Your specialist subject

> *First you must know your chosen subject well. With commitment to learning about an area of interest, anyone can become a mastermind of knowledge and expertise, and to develop their interest to become an expert in their own field. It is useful to gain a broad knowledge base, including both the clinical and social perspectives of the condition, to get the full picture.* (JULIA QUICKFALL)

There may be no question about this. Maybe, as a midwife working with very young parents, you are clear that this is your subject and your passion. It is the care of, and services for, these young people that you want to influence. Becoming known as an informal expert in this area will give you the platform to do this.

But suppose, as a hospital pharmacist, you have a wide range of different responsibilities with several areas of special interest. You have a general aim to 'get on', to become known in your profession, and to influence the way pharmacy services are used and pharmacists are perceived. What topic do you choose to become expert in? The potential choices are:

- *breadth or depth?* Will you become a voice on pharmacy issues generally, or a commentator on the details of the use of robotics in dispensing?
- *precise or general?* Will you deal in the technical details of robotic systems, or the training implications of increasing technology to streamline hospital systems?
- *new or established area?* Other people have written about robotics – will you build on this, or find a completely new topic like automatic dispensing via ATMs (by the time you read this, it may not be a new subject . . .)?
- *fixed or fluid?* Will you always write about robotics in pharmacy (so making it worth investing in courses, books and site visits), or move onto your other areas of interest in due course?

Even someone with an apparently clear and very specialist role in their professional life can make the sort of choices outlined above, by combining different elements of their work in different ways. An example of options for a 'specialist subject' for a physiotherapist, working part-time in a private sports clinic and part-time for a local football club, and specialising in ankle sprains, is shown in Table 15.1.

TABLE 15.1 Options for 'specialist subjects' for a sports injury physiotherapist working both in private practice and for a football club, and specialising in ankle injuries

Aspect of work – focus on:	Acute treatment	Rehabilitation	Private practice	Sports clinics	Football club	Youth work	Patient education
Physiotherapy career options			X		X		
Working with the community						X	X
Working in an inner city area				X		X	
Sports jobs	X	X		X	X		
Working with footballers	X	X			X	X	
Dealing with ankle injuries	X						X

Each X in a box represents a potential article for this practitioner to write. The 16 different articles could be targeted at a wide range of journals: from specialist physiotherapy journals (about careers and private practice), to general nursing journals (working with the community, patient information), specialist nursing journals (for practice nurses, accident and emergency (A&E) nurses) and community care journals (youth work, patient education, working with football clubs)

Your chosen topic may be professional or service related rather than clinical, of course. Subjects such as the use of complementary therapies in your field, staff training, the relevant benefits system, evidence-based practice, and professional regulation are of perennial interest. Or there may be another element of your life that is important to you, and that you would use to take a particular perspective on your work – such as multiculturalism, spirituality or sexuality.

MIRROR MOMENT

Think honestly about why you want to become an expert. If your principal motivation is to make a name for yourself and enhance your career, focus on two or three topics that will give you the widest possible reach and broaden the range of opportunities likely to come your way. Pick those that are topical, but look as if they might last – if possible, something that is new in your profession and few people are currently writing or speaking about. Be prepared to drop a subject and move on if necessary.

If your principal motivation is influencing the agenda on a specific cause, focus on in-depth knowledge of this subject. You will need a wide range of knowledge about it, as well as depth, so that you can write and speak from different perspectives – otherwise your opportunities to influence will be limited. Be prepared to adapt your message, and change the way you present it, to keep it fresh.

Three phases of informal expertise

These can be classed as:

- preparation
- starting out
- maintaining your expertise.

Preparation

> *Always be willing to say 'will try' not 'can't be done.' I would also say be prepared to move out of your comfort zone to do things – people notice a tryer.* (JUDITH WHITTAM)

Before beginning to build expertise on a specific topic or topics, it would be very beneficial to:

- *read a wider range of journals, in practice, research and management*: to see what they say about your subject and to spot opportunities to write an article, submit a conference abstract, or respond to a letter
- *join an email discussion group*: to find the names of interested people on the subject, test their views on ideas you have, and find inspiration for new things to write or say about your subject
- *use online abstract searching facilities*: the quickest way to see what has been published on your subject, get references and find other experts
- *keep hard copy reference files*: it saves a lot of time when you are preparing an article, a presentation or a letter if you have the key documents relevant to your subject in one place, as you will be constantly quoting and referencing them (*see* Box 15.1 for the kinds of things you could usefully keep to hand in these files)
- *make sure you have full copies of key documents*: rather than relying on summary documents, or a journalist's analysis in their weekly journal, for information on major policy and research developments. By reading the original in full, you will automatically have more information to draw on for articles, speeches or presentations. Read it once carefully, and make notes or use a highlighter pen to save you going over it repeatedly
- *find the relevant policy contacts*: look on the websites of government departments to find names on relevant policy documents (*see* Box 15.2) so that you can make contact in due course
- *check regularly for new books on your subject*: use online book stores, health book publishers' websites, the book review column of your journals and your local medical library – buy or borrow them and at least skim read so that you know who is saying what, and who publishes what, so you can spot opportunities to propose a new book, or chapter in a book

- having found the other 'names' in your field, as authors, researchers, policy makers or speakers, start to make contact and build them into your network – the next time they have to turn down an invitation to write a piece, speak to a journalist or present at a study day, and they are asked to suggest someone else (organisers and editors are cunning that way) they may think of you.

BOX 15.1 Hard copy reference files: useful content

- The latest policy documents on the subject
- Relevant National Service Frameworks, National Institute for Health and Clinical Excellence (NICE) guidance or other service specification designed for long-term use
- Major research studies
- Major background documents
- Information leaflets or briefings from professional organisations, relevant charities or patient groups
- Key articles

BOX 15.2 Government departments with relevant information

- *Department of Health*: on health and social care, NHS and independent sector
- *Department for Education and Skills*: for children's services, nurseries, 'early years' work with children, child protection
- *Home Office*: for issues related to crime, violence, social disorder, refugees and asylum seekers, justice
- *Department for Work and Pensions*: for welfare issues, child poverty, carers, sickness certification, disability, rehabilitation
- *Cabinet Office*: on emergency planning, and regulation of the public sector
- *Office of the Deputy Prime Minister*: for issues of regional government, homelessness, social exclusion, business support and regional development agencies

Note: the responsibilities of government departments may be changed during cabinet 'reshuffles' – always check the relevant websites to be sure which department is responsible for any issue you are interested in.

Starting out

> *Avoid jargon and management gobbledegook – it may sound impressive at first, but leads to confusion. Be grounded in reality – you need to know what is happening 'on the ground' to make robust proposals.* (JUDY HARGADON)

- *Writing*: start by responding to articles relevant to your subject with a letter, or by offering the editor a comment piece with an alternative view or a different perspective on the subject. At the same time, you could write to the author of the piece with a comment or compliment – it is always possible to be positive and enthusiastic, even if your view is quite different – to make the link with them. Talk to the editor of the journal you know best about writing an article for them – this is always a better approach than submitting 'cold' (*see* Chapter 17 for more on writing for publication). The sooner you are in print, the sooner your reputation on the subject will take root.

- *Towards book chapters*: a good way to start getting involved with books is by reviewing them. For a start, it will usually get you a free copy of the book. And your name will become associated in the editor's and readers' mind with the topic on which you review, which will make you more likely to be asked to write a chapter in future. The process of reading and reviewing books will also give you ideas for different structures and approaches you can take to writing for a book. But it is important to make the reviews meaningful and intelligent – anyone can re-hash the publisher's blurb and the foreword into a couple of hundred words, but this will not fool editors. Make sure you have something useful to say about the book.
- *Conferences*: put in an abstract for a conference. A workshop or poster presentation is a better place to start than a platform presentation – which are often by invitation rather than offer. But the opportunities that arise from workshop and poster presentations can be as important as from giving a 'big speech', since you will be able to engage in dialogue with interested people, exchange contacts, and build your networks, as well as exposing your name and expertise to a wide group of people. *See* Chapter 10 on getting the most out of attending conferences, and Chapter 22 for more on using conferences to influence.
- *Other speaking opportunities*: you don't have to hold out for a major national conference to raise your profile as an expert on a topic. At the beginning, it is worth accepting every opportunity to speak: to local professional groups, patient groups, meetings, journal clubs. Each one is a chance to practise your presentation skills, to indicate your interest to a new set of people, and to refine your knowledge a little more. If you are properly prepared, speak with confidence within the bounds of your knowledge, and make clear that you are happy to learn as well as to share; then every 'appearance', however small or informal the group, will build your reputation.

PORTFOLIO POINTER

Remember to record every 'event' at which you present in your portfolio, including the size and nature of the group, the exact topic or angle on which you spoke, and the nature of your presentation. Speaker's forms for submitting conference abstracts often ask about your experience, and being able to produce an (honest) list will reassure them that you are able to talk to a group, you know how to prepare and tailor your material for different occasions, and you are not likely to freeze on the spot or duck out at the last minute.

- *Creating your own opportunities*: if you are not being invited to speak about your topic, think about creating your own opportunities to do so. These could range from putting on your own local or regional study day (with other speakers as well), to offering an update on the topic to staff in your own work area. Whatever you do, bear in mind your responsibility to know your topic, be honest about what you can offer, prepare meticulously and deliver well. Becoming an expert is not about fooling people, but about taking the first steps to develop yourself as a genuine resource on your subject.

PERSONAL DEVELOPMENT EXERCISE

When you have developed an area of special interest, and begun to write and speak about it, be sure to update your CV to include reference to it. It is the kind of additional enterprise and effort that makes one candidate stand out from the crowd of others.

Maintaining your expertise

> *One of the commonest mistakes people make is not evolving their ideas when others have good things to input: the best ideas are a compound. Lots of people feel too much ownership of an idea and will not change it because of that.* (SANDRA MELLORS)

There are some people who develop a niche in a particular subject, then continue to say the same thing in much the same way for years. Most of us have encountered the person who will 'give his talk on X' every year to every new group of students, or inductees, with the same slides, regardless of relevance, and heedless of changing evidence or practice. And this bad habit is not confined to any one profession.

> *Be careful not to get branded – you may feel strongly about something, but if you always go on about it, you will lose impact on other issues.* (JUDY HARGADON)

It is vital, to maintain your reputation, that you are seen to remain credible, interesting and authoritative over time. These are some of the things you can do to ensure that this is the case:

- *keep up with the latest policy documents and statements*: keep the relevant websites, of government departments, professional associations, relevant charities and pressure groups, on your 'Favourites' list, and check them regularly for new information: you don't want to be talking about the draft document, or consultation version, once the final version is out
- *keep up with the latest jargon on the subject*: however much we deride 'spin' and 'political correctness', nothing sounds quite as out of touch as last month's name for something. If diabetes in young people is your thing, you should know whether

it is currently referred to as 'juvenile onset' or 'type 1' or 'insulin dependent' – or something else entirely. Professions Allied to Medicine changed to Allied Health Professionals several years ago, and reference to 'PAMs' now jars audiences noticeably – but still happens

- *use your growing reputation to approach more senior people in your profession or clinical interest group*: when you can say 'I'm running a workshop on coronary angioplasty at a conference next month . . .', or 'I'm updating my regional forum on new developments in pharmacy', you have the perfect reason to contact others in the field for information, advice or examples – and add them to your active network
- *start to be choosy about opportunities*: once you have a reputation to maintain, you can begin to choose the bigger, better platforms for your expertise. This does not mean ignoring other requests, or even refusing them politely – sometimes it might be politic to speak to the small local group – but unless you have unlimited time out from your day job, you may need to prioritise. This is where your network can pay dividends, as you may be able to help out the organisers of events that you turn down by suggesting an alternative speaker, building goodwill for yourself in both parties in the process
- *always respond to requests for help or information from others*: this network building works both ways. While you are contacting more senior people for their expertise, others who are less experienced in the field, or experienced but with less profile, will be contacting you for your expertise. It should always be possible to respond to them, and offer something helpful. Your reputation will benefit – and conversely, it will suffer if you become known as someone who is happy to speak at conferences, but never responds to individuals. This looks as if you are more interested in self-promotion than sharing professional expertise
- *also respond to criticisms*: one of the inevitable outcomes of raising your head above the professional parapet is that someone will shoot at it. Unless a letter or email is downright abusive, it is usually better to respond than to ignore it. You can be sure the writer will not say to their circle 'I sent this abusive email and he just ignored it'. They will say 'I wrote to him after the conference, but he didn't even bother to reply'. So do reply – but briefly, neutrally and politely. *See* Chapter 26 for 'coping with the consequences' of your power to influence
- *keep your material as well as your knowledge fresh*: always look for a different angle, a new quote, or a better way of presenting data, and update your presentation. Check that organisations' names haven't changed (it seems to happen every few months in the NHS), and that your slides don't have the name of the last conference at which you spoke on the title slide. Keep it fresh physically as well: no dusty old acetates, or outdated PowerPoint® backgrounds, or dodgy floppy disks when everyone else is using memory sticks, or the latest technology.

Developing a reputation as an expert on your topic of interest really is as simple as this. The only reason that the NHS world is not overflowing with experts – and if it was, we wouldn't see the same names at conferences, in journals and on books over and over again – is that many people don't have the motivation, and so don't make the time, to turn themselves into experts. If you want to, you can.

MIRROR MOMENT

Do you want to do this? Notice it is motivation, not time, that comes first in the sentence above. Time is elastic and can always be stretched to accommodate the things you really want to do. Motivation is the key. It doesn't matter what that motivation is, but if you have it, recognise it, and start building yourself up as an expert now.

Top tips

Remember these top tips for 'expertise-building':

- display enthusiasm, not arrogance
- helping others is good for your reputation
- some responses and contacts you get will be negative – deal with them well to enhance your reputation
- keep up with developments, including language, to protect your credibility
- keep your presentation materials and methods fresh.

PERSONAL DEVELOPMENT EXERCISE

Find yourself two opportunities in the next six months to build your reputation in your chosen areas: they could be articles, speaking opportunities, letters to journals or other outlets. Record them in your portfolio so that you can use them in future.

CHECKLIST FOR ACTION

Have you:

- decided which topic(s) you will build your expertise and reputation on: something you are genuinely interested and enthusiastic about?
- planned what kind of opportunities you will look for?
- started to explore information on websites and in policy documents on your chosen topic(s)?

CHAPTER 16

Entering for awards

If you are in doubt about the suitability of your application for the award, always check. Contact the awards administrator before you start completing your application. They are always happy to talk things through and it saves them and you a great deal of time and effort. (ANNE PEARSON)

It is astonishingly difficult to give awards to healthcare professionals. Not because there are no good ones, or none doing good work, but because, in my experience, they are generally so reluctant to enter themselves or their work into the process. 'I couldn't possibly enter for a national award', 'We wouldn't stand a chance' or 'We're nothing special' are the common explanations. However, this is very often not the case.

Giving awards

As an example: the Queen's Nursing Institute had more than 500 enquiries about a set of awards that offered £15,000 funding for community-based projects focused on any aspect of public health or long-term conditions. A total of just 36 completed applications were received, of which 28 were eligible. We had funding for four projects, so at this stage – assuming equal quality of proposals – every applicant had a one in seven chance of success. We interviewed the eight project teams with the most exciting ideas and best applications: they had a one in two chance of being funded.

The many organisations I have worked with who run awards schemes for health professionals all share this experience. They have too few applicants, and too few good-quality applications, for most rounds of awards. Sometimes these schemes have to defer closing dates, re-advertise or lower the quality bar and make awards to almost everyone who applies, simply in order to avoid cancelling the whole scheme. It shouldn't come to this – there is good work, and there are excellent practitioners, that deserve recognition, reward, and funding to put their projects into place or their research into action.

This chapter aims to help you access the funding, profile and opportunities for influence that come with awards. As with many other activities described in this book, the secret is that there is no secret! It is not difficult to make a successful application for an award, yet many people shy away from trying, and many of those who do try make elementary mistakes or oversights that cost them success. Doing the simple things right will make it very likely that you will succeed.

Why bother?

Entering for an award in a way that is going to impress the judges takes time and effort. It is an addition to your day to day work, and may require thinking through your ideas, talking to new people, researching the topic, testing the waters with others, getting permissions, finding out costs . . . It is not something that can be lost in the daily round. So what could be in it for you? There are three main types of award:

- *funding awards*: there are different awards that provide money to finance a project, a research study, a course or equipment for the winner. They focus on investing in your skills and ideas, so generally require a clear exposition of the benefits that will accrue to you as a professional, your patients, service or organisation as a result of winning the award
- *recognition awards*: these awards are retrospective rather than prospective, and designed to reward and publicise good practice, innovative services or effective change. Examples are 'Team of the Year' and 'Public Servant of the Year'-type awards. The award is often tangible – a trophy or certificate – but these awards may also give some money to the winner, either as a personal 'prize', or for them to spend on training or equipment for the workplace. They are generally looking for clear evidence of the outcomes of the work being presented, in terms of benefits for patients, improved services or better working practices
- *opportunity awards*: other awards, such as fellowships, travel bursaries and scholarships, provide a chance to make a visit, or carry out a study, to fulfil a specific aim. They are also very useful as pivots for career change. For these, organisers are looking for a very specific purpose, a clear plan for achieving it, and often a commitment to provide a report, speech or lecture at the end of the agreed time.

The connections between entering for awards and having influence are very powerful – *see* Box 16.1 for a summary. In addition to the benefits listed above, just *entering* for an award brings you, your work and your enthusiasm to the attention of a new set of people, often in national organisations. As well as the administrators of the awards, there are likely to be judges who are specialists in your field, and funders for the awards who have national reach and influence. In preparing your application, you will be connecting with new people in your own organisation, and learning about functions you may not normally have access to, such as finance and communications.

If you win an award, of course, your profile will automatically be enhanced, giving you more opportunities to influence. All the professional journals cover awards schemes, and, as they are always hungry for articles about something new, there are ready-made opportunities for articles, interviews and letters. Award ceremonies always get good coverage – and they are good places to rub shoulders with a new set of influential contacts. Some awards bring their own specific professional opportunities: for example, the winner of Practice Nurse of the Year is automatically invited to sit on the editorial board of the *Practice Nurse* journal. And all awards are an asset to your CV: no matter how local or small-scale, they show that you have had the enthusiasm and commitment to put together an entry, and do something worthy of funding or reward. At national level – where you are just as likely to succeed – they have even greater impact.

BOX 16.1 How entering for awards gains you influence

- By introducing you to judges who are experts in your field
- By putting you in contact with national organisations
- By providing the opportunity to mix with people from other parts of the UK working in the same field on a course or award programme
- By giving you material from your project, research or travel to write and speak about
- By providing publicity that will bring other contacts to you
- By raising your profile as an innovator and/or leader
- By giving you practice at presenting your case for change in writing and, often, at interview
- By giving you specific opportunities to speak in public about your work

So entering awards is a win–win: there are the benefits for your patients, service, organisation and career if you win; and benefits for your influence and networking even if you don't.

MIRROR MOMENT

Stop and think about what kind of award you are interested in. If it is principally for your career benefit, you may focus on scholarships and bursaries. If you have an idea you want to implement to influence practice, look for the funding awards. If you want to raise your profile, or promote your unit, the retrospective '. . . of the Year' awards are probably most suitable. It doesn't matter what your motivation is – but it does affect the award you choose and the nature of your application, so it is counter-productive to kid yourself!

Making an application

Don't assume that the person who reviews your application knows you, your specialty or the area in which you work. Paint a picture of what you are doing – if possible, ask someone unconnected with your area of work to read through your application – do they understand what you want to do?
(Anne Pearson)

The whole process – from finding the right award to the judge's decision – can be undertaken in a logical, stepwise manner that helps integrate it with your other work. This approach can also highlight opportunities to involve other people at different stages, so sharing the burden between you.

Ten steps to success in awards

Step 1: Find out what is available

The least effective – but depressingly common – ways to find an award scheme to enter are:

- working up an idea then searching for somewhere to send it
- emailing random people in national organisations to ask if they have any money.

A much better approach is to research organisations that offer awards through their websites – where you will be able to check eligibility criteria, closing dates, information required in an application and other essential data. Many websites will allow you download the application form and guidance notes, and later submit the application electronically. Alternatively, you can search via a website specifically designed to pull together information about awards available from a range of sources, such as rdinfo.org.uk and rdfunding.org.uk, which will identify some places you might never have thought to look. Some of the available websites are shown in Box 16.2.

BOX 16.2 Websites to search for information on awards

- www.rdfunding.org.uk: this database currently holds information from 1,354 funding bodies offering 5,641 different awards
- The Queen's Nursing Institute: www.qni.org.uk
- The Foundation for Nursing Studies: www.fons.org
- The Florence Nightingale Foundation: www.florence-nightingale-foundation.org.uk
- The Burdett Trust for Nursing: www.burdettnursingtrust.org.uk
- The Worshipful Company of Curriers: www.curriers.co.uk
- The Health Foundation: www.health.org.uk

For the retrospective, 'reward' awards, watch for advertisements in the various professional and management journals, as well as relevant health and social care sections of the quality press. These awards take place all year, but with a preponderance of closing dates in summer, ready for autumn award ceremonies. Read the widest range of journals you can, and if it is a team award you have in mind, make sure different disciplines within the team are checking the journals they read.

It is important not to limit yourself to looking at health-related charities and organisations for awards: opportunities can turn up much further afield. For example, the Worshipful Company of Curriers in London – one of the craftsmen's guilds in the leather industry – offers substantial awards to health professionals whose work will benefit people living in the City of London.

PERSONAL DEVELOPMENT EXERCISE

Think about a specific project that you would like to carry out in your area of work, or a research project you would like to undertake; then look for at least two organisations that might fund it. Even if you are not ready to apply now, it is a useful exercise to know where you might go.

Step 2: Find the right kind of award

If you have thought about what you want from an award you will know what kind of award you are looking for. Select these out of the range you have found on websites and in journals, to narrow down your search. It is also worth contacting these organisations to ask if they know of any other organisations offering similar types of award: many award-making bodies will know each other's criteria and schemes very well and could point you to similar bodies that you may not have heard of. If you don't want to ask by email or telephone (and so alert them that you are looking around), then check their website links for similar organisations.

Step 3: Find the award that is the 'best fit' with you, your team or your project

This will not only make it easier for you to put together your application – because you all speak the same professional language – but will increase your chances of success by limiting the competition. For example, as a health visitor, you could enter a wide range of award schemes open to health professionals, public health workers, community workers or similar. But this opens up the competition. If you target an award limited to health visitors, you will greatly reduce the number of potential entrants. If you find an award for health visitors working in the field of domestic violence, you will thin out the competition even further. Such precisely targeted awards are not uncommon, partly because awards are often sponsored by a company or trust fund with very specific interests.

'Best fit' should include matters such as timescale: if the research funding is to be made available over three years, and you want to do a course in one year, the award is not suitable. Similarly, travel scholarships often specify a date by which the travel has to take place: check that this does not conflict with your career or family plans.

Bear in mind also that some awards have geographical restrictions, and are only open to people working in a specific place. This clearly adds another limiter to the crowd of applicants, but *see* below . . .

Step 4: Check that what is on offer matches your needs

In finding the 'best fit' award, make sure you haven't sacrificed the reason you wanted to enter in the first place. If the award for a health visitor working in domestic violence in Surrey provides funding for a project, and funding is what you want, this is not a problem. But if what you wanted was to raise your personal profile nationally in the field of adult protection, this may not be as effective as entering for a national award. On the other hand, funding that enables you to run your local project will give you something to write about in the national journals, and speak about at the conferences, that will get you national attention.

Step 5: Make your decision on the award you will enter

This is the pivot point: from now on, you are targeting a specific award and awarding body, and everything you do should aim to maximise your chances with that specific organisation. In making your decision, consider the nature of the relationship you will have with the funder. Some want frequent reports and/or regular site visits. Some just want a final report. Some expect you to be available for a lot of publicity, or to give a lecture at the end of your award period, or attend a gala dinner. These things are not meant to be negotiable: this is 'what's in it for them'. If you can't meet their expectations, don't enter for their award.

Conversely, look also at what's in it for you apart from the award. Will you get professional development, help and advice, skills training or assistance to publish? These are valuable elements that form part of the two-way relationship you will have with the funding organisation.

Step 6: Get all the information available on the award and awarding organisation

You need to know:

- *what are the stated aims of the award*: so you can be sure that your application shows how you or your team or project will meet them
- *who is eligible to enter*: including how many people can be in the team, and whether they can or should be from different professions, or include patient or service user representatives
- *what limits there are on the topic, scope or size of a project, or of the work you can enter for recognition*: how long ago can work have happened, or be planned to happen, and still be eligible?
- *the closing date for entries* (enough time to prepare a good application?) and the timeframe for the delivering the project or report, or undertaking the research or study trip (realistic in view of other commitments?)
- *background on the organisation offering the award*: its aims, scope, influence and affiliations – it may receive its award funding from a source you consider unethical, or from one with a specific interest that you can target in your application. Simply demonstrating some knowledge and appreciation of the organisation's history, aims and values during the application process will create a good impression
- *the process involved in entering the award*: what forms you need to complete, how you should submit them, what kind of evidence or references will be needed, and so on. You may need to submit a written entry only, or travel across the country to be interviewed. The organisation may or may not offer travel expenses for attending interviews. Some awards involve judges coming to visit you on-site to see your work or interview you. Some awards involve publicity for short-listed

applicants – are you (and your organisation) prepared to be photographed and written about regardless of whether you ultimately win an award?

- *who judges the award*: these are key people whom you will want to impress, and it is better to know in advance who is involved so that you can prepare your material and yourself appropriately (*see* Box 16.3 for a salutary tale).

BOX 16.3 Preparing to meet the judges: a cautionary tale

I sat on the judging panel for awards being made by the Worshipful Company of Curriers in London. The name of the organisation, the history described on its website and the venue for interviews – Apothecaries' Hall in the City – should have given the applicants some clues as to the nature of the interviews. The panel consisted of seven people, including the Master of the Company, the Past Master, the President and the Clerk of the Company, and took place in the Grand Hall. The award applicants, some of whom were very casually dressed and clearly had not anticipated the questions or rehearsed any answers, were visibly intimidated and uncomfortable. They put themselves at an unnecessary disadvantage by not having anticipated the formality of the interviews.

Very often, all of this information is supplied to you in an application pack. If not, much of it will be easily available on the organisation's website. If you need more, contact the awarding body directly by telephone or email: be polite, focused and business-like, as these calls are often noted and form part of the file on your application when you submit it. They create an impression of you: 'Called to ask for paper copy of form as doesn't know how to download it' doesn't help if your project application involves any degree of IT use at all!

Other useful information to be found on websites includes details of previous winners, their projects, studies or reports. These can give you an idea of the kind of projects that have succeeded before, and where there are gaps you could fill.

Step 7: Make sure you are ready before starting the application form

If it is a retrospective award, you may need to check that others who were involved in the work are willing to be included, and that your organisation is aware of it at all the right levels such as managers and press office. You will need outcome or evaluation data to show what was good about it, and you might need to line up referees who will back your application. If a site visit is part of the judging process, you will need to know that you can get permission for this, from managers, staff and patients.

If it is a prospective award for a project or study trip, check:

- do you have all the necessary people 'on board'? These are the people you need to help you deliver the project or research, or cover your post while you are away – there is no point winning the funding if you are then prevented from doing anything with it. Make sure you have permission to proceed, if needed
- is anyone likely to sabotage your plans? Is so, can you win them over by including them, keeping them informed, showing how the award could benefit them or their work?

- can you meet the timescale?
- how will you or your organisation handle the funding if it comes in, and the publicity? It is best not to spring these things on finance or communications departments as a *fait accompli*
- have you involved patients in your plan for this project or study? Many awarding organisations look for evidence of professionals and patients working together.

Step 8: Complete the application

> *Make sure that your evaluation measures reflect your aims and objectives – that they will provide evidence of impact.* (ANNE PEARSON)

It is the simple things that defeat many people, and simply following the instructions for completion and submission of the application form will greatly endear you to the judges. Leave plenty of time for last minute hitches, including time to show it to others locally and respond to their comments. Try to submit by email, if this is the organisation's preference, or by post (watch out for 'by midday on . . .' instructions). Although some places accept faxed applications, these inevitably give the impression of a last minute rush and lack of organisation, which will not help you.

Do send all the documentation requested: having to chase up CVs or references creates unnecessary work for the awarding organisation, and they would be entitled to dismiss your application as incomplete, so wasting all the work you have put in. Also make sure you send the number of copies requested. See Box 16.4 for tips on creating a CV to back up an award application.

BOX 16.4 Creating a CV to back an award application

Key tips:

- keep it short (2 pages maximum): this is not a job application
- only include relevant information: the judges don't need to know about your O levels, hobbies or children
- show that you have a history of taking on projects or study in addition to your day job
- show that you complete things you start
- give specific examples of your previous innovative work, study or interest in other places, as appropriate to the award you are entering
- use facts and figures to demonstrate that you understand, believe in, and can do, outcome evaluation.

Step 9: Make the best of the interview or site visit

Whether you go to them, or they come to you, there are some simple ways to impress the awards judging panel:

- know the organisation's and the judges' backgrounds and show you have bothered to find out (without telling them things they already know about their organisation)

- smile, relax and talk to all of them
- use lots of facts, figures and outcome measures
- make it easy for them – they may be interviewing a lot of people or teams – by being succinct and using visual aids sparingly
- let them see your enthusiasm and your passion – it tends to be infectious.

If judges come to you on a site visit, do look after them with at least basic courtesy. I once went out to a site as a judge to find that we were crammed into a small clinic room, kept waiting for the award nominee, interrupted by phone calls when talking to her, given unwieldy sandwiches with no plate, loaded up with bulky examples of the work to carry home, and finally left to find our own way out of the building and back to the railway station. Looking after people is not so much a matter of buttering up the judges (though surely it crossed their minds that it couldn't hurt?) as simple good manners! The judges are very likely to be expert and influential people in a field relevant to yours: whether or not you gain the award, this is an opportunity to impress them.

Step 10: Handling the outcome

If you are successful, you should of course thank all the people in your organisation who were involved in the application, as co-applicants, supporters, referees, or managers. This will smooth the way for the difficult delivery bit ahead! You will also need to let the finance and communications people know that they should swing into action in their respective ways.

If you are not successful, see if the awarding body will give you feedback on your application – some will but some can't. Review the application yourself to see what can be learned from it. Perhaps it was unrealistic, vague on costings, or poorly presented? Start looking for a different opportunity to submit the work or idea – after you have revised the application to fit the new funder's requirements, of course. Again, thank everyone who helped along the way, and keep them updated on your next moves.

PORTFOLIO POINTER

Keep a copy of any award applications you make, even if they are not successful. They will contain useful summary CV and other information you might want to lift out in future; and you can use the fact that you entered as an illustration of your enterprise and energy when applying for future jobs.

The commonest mistakes in applying for awards

These are, in my experience:

- an over-ambitious idea
- going it alone when a team would be more likely to deliver

- applying to the wrong source for the work you want to enter
- poorly prepared and presented application forms
- excessive jargon and generalities
- exaggerated claims for potential outcomes.

Finally, remember that winning an award is only the start of the relationship with your funding body. You will now need to build those links to get the most out of your award.

CHECKLIST FOR ACTION

Have you:

- identified the kind of award you are interested in?
- searched the web for organisations that fund this kind of award?
- visited their websites for details and forms?

CHAPTER 17

Writing for publication

> *The most important thing for a new writer is that you must have something to say to the reader. A good writing style alone will not get you published – good ideas are as important, if not more so.* (JEAN GRAY)

Having an article published in a professional journal or magazine is one of the easiest ways to reach and influence large numbers of people who work in the same area of care as you. Many more people will read an article than will ever hear you speak at a conference. It is also a very effective way of getting your name in front of national organisations and policy makers, and building a reputation that will generate invitations to join project groups or advisory forums. As Chapter 15 explained, it is relatively easy to establish yourself as an expert in a particular subject, and one of the main mechanisms is through writing articles.

Yet for many practitioners, the idea of writing something for publication is daunting, and the process of getting it published is a mystery. This section aims to demonstrate a simple, step-by-step approach to getting an article published.

Myths and truths

Before beginning the process of publication, it is worth dealing with some persistent myths, and facing some hard truths. Amongst the most prevalent myths is the idea that you have to be really good at writing to get published. This is not the case – journals are staffed by people who are very good at fine-tuning and improving prose. That is their job. What they need from you is the idea, project, debate, idea or description of your work that their readers will be interested in. If you follow the steps suggested below, you can be 80–90% sure of getting your article published, no matter how ordinary your writing skills.

Another dangerous myth is that you can simply write down your material then 'send it on the rounds' to the journals. This is a time-wasting and soul-destroying route to unpublished obscurity. Much better to take the preliminary steps of finding the right journal, and checking that the editor is interested in your idea, before you start writing.

Equally bad practice, but still too common, is writing an article and sending it to several journals at once, in the hope that one of them will publish it. Apart from the fact that this means it cannot possibly be well-suited to most of the journals, since they all have different requirements, the editors will be extremely annoyed if more than one of them wants it and you have to give it to one and withdraw it from another. Your reputation as a writer will be badly damaged and they will not want to deal with you again.

Some other myths to be disposed of are:

- *'You have to write about something really amazing'*: not so. There is very little that is really new or unique in health and social care: but you should aim to have a different view, a new approach, something challenging to say or some topical reason for writing about your subject
- *'The journals must be swamped with articles, they won't want mine'*: some journals do receive a lot of submissions, but many of these make elementary mistakes, are wrongly targeted or unsuitable for other reasons. No editor I have ever spoken to has an excess of interesting, well-presented, appropriately tailored articles for every issue. There is room for yours!
- *'It's not worth writing for the weekly 'comics'*: except that they have huge readerships! For all that people sometimes disparage them, these are the magazines that most people read, so give you the widest audience for your piece
- *'If the article is rejected, it's obviously not good enough . . . I can't write'*: this is not the case. Articles are rejected for many reasons other than the quality of the writing, and most of these rejections can be avoided by following the steps described below.

Hard facts

Disposing of the myths is encouraging – but there are some facts to face as well.

It is important to accept that your material has to fit the publication, not the other way round. If they take articles of 2,000 words, they are not going to publish your thesis of 10,000 words, even cut down by half, no matter how good it is. Similarly, if they publish research findings, they will not be interested in your opinion piece on the state of social work training.

It is also important to remember that journals exist to benefit the publishers and the careers of the editorial team, not the cause of patients, clients or even professionals. So they may choose to publish your incautious views, dangerous sense of humour or demolition of local decision making, because it makes for a good controversy that will keep the letters page busy for weeks. You cannot expect them to protect you or your career by advising you to think again about your piece.

Finally, an encouraging fact, often disbelieved: if you receive a request to revise or amend your article, this is not a rejection! It is in fact a conditional acceptance. Do the revision, even though it is more work, because the editor would not go to the trouble of inviting you to do so, and waiting patiently for the revised version, if they did not intend to use it.

Steps to publication

> *The best advice I can give to potential authors is to read the magazine you want to write for: most magazines have their own format and will not publish an article that does not fit, except in highly unusual circumstances.*
> (JEAN GRAY)

The main steps on the way to getting an article published are shown in Figure 17.1. Note that 80% of the process happens before you start writing: this is the largest part of ensuring you will be published, and it doesn't involve any writing skills at all!

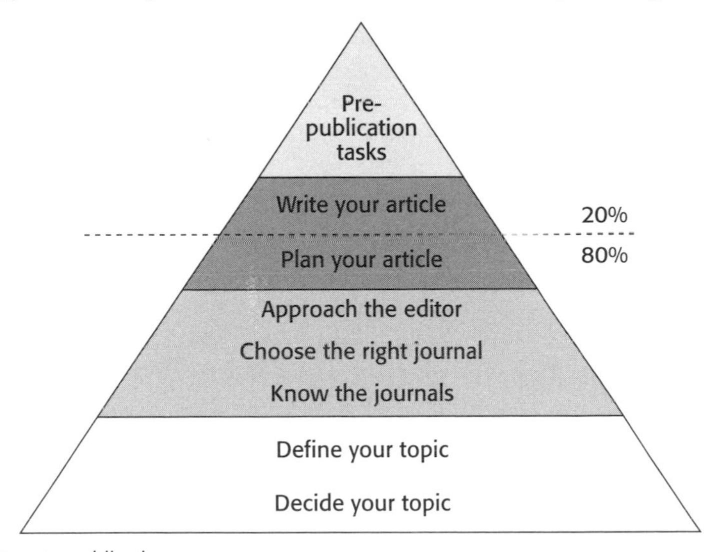

Figure 17.1 Steps to publication

Step 1: Decide your topic

You may have something quite specific in mind – a piece of work, an opinion or some particular expertise to share. Or you may just want to write anything in order to build your profile, but not be sure what. That decision – or identification of your specific idea – is your starting point.

Step 2: Define your topic

This is a much more detailed process that has to be thought through before you go any further. You cannot find the right journal, much less have a useful conversation with an editor, without knowing the answer to three key questions:

- what *exactly* is the article going to be about?
- who is it aimed at?
- why should they be reading it?

Suppose you have been running a project, and your decision at step 1 was that you want to write about this work. There are still decisions to be made about which aspect of the work you focus on, who your target audience is and whether you write it to inform the reader of interesting findings, to warn them of pitfalls, to encourage them to replicate the work or to debate a professional issue that has arisen during the project. Figure 17.2 uses a real project to illustrate the different answers you could arrive at in considering the first of these questions.

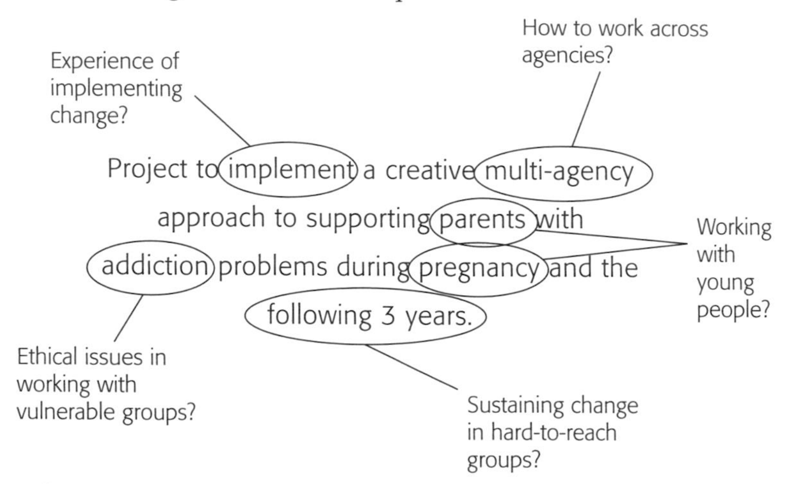

Figure 17.2 What exactly will you write about?

Step 3: Know the journals

To find the right place for the type of article you want to write, you need to know the key characteristics of a range of journals. It is easy to focus only on the one you read most frequently, and which you already know well – but this may not help if they are unlikely to publish the kind of article you have in mind. If you want to write up the detailed statistical analysis you carried out at the start of the project, your weekly magazine-type practitioner journal is probably not going to be interested. Conversely, if you want to illustrate the impact of your project on the service users, using their stories and photographs, a research-focused title is not going to accept your article. The same distinction applies to your identified readership. If you want to address social workers, you will aim for a different journal than if you hope to influence midwives. So you need to get to know a wider range of journals, and you need to know some quite precise things about them (*see* Box 17.1). The easiest way to do this is to use a library or resource centre, rather than buying journals. This allows you to look at two or three back copies as well as the current issue. Or you can borrow from colleagues, check websites or pick up free copies at conferences.

BOX 17.1 Assessing the journals

For each journal, check:

- *the aim:*
  - what does the journal say its aims are: publishing research, keeping practitioners up to date, speaking for a particular group, linking different groups, lobbying for change?

- who does it say it is aimed at? This will often appear under the title, or on the page with staff names and contact details. Does it identify itself by the care group it is focused on (the elderly, people with diabetes, mothers) or the professionals/workers it wants to reach (health visitors, doctors, social workers)?
- *the staff/writers*: who edits it? Are there section editors? These will be on the page with contact details, address etc. What kind of authors are they publishing (this should be at the top or bottom of the article)?
- *submissions*: what do the guidelines for authors say? Are they published in the journal or do you need to send for them/see them on the website?
- *type of articles*: do they publish opinion pieces? Research papers? Descriptive articles? Clinical updates? Discussion pieces? Educational pieces – with or without self-assessments attached?
- *format of articles*: do they have boxes, photographs and bullet points? Do they follow a particular format? Do they include tables, graphs and illustrations? How long are they?

It is vital that you do look at the latest issue of the journal as well, not only ones from several weeks or months ago: people move on, formats change and new topics are covered – unless you are absolutely up to date, you could embarrass yourself and waste a lot of time approaching the wrong person or journal with your idea.

PERSONAL DEVELOPMENT EXERCISE

Find four different journals to assess using the questions in Box 17.1. Mix your own profession's or area of work's journals with some read by colleagues from a different area of healthcare, to see how different they are. If you work in social care, include a health-focused journal, and vice versa. While you have them to hand, photocopy the guidelines for authors – these are essential before you start to write.

Step 4: Choose the right journal

With a wider knowledge of the kinds of publications around, you should be able to identify a journal likely to be interested in the article you want to write, and that is read by the kind of people you would like to speak to. You need to match the content, audience and purpose of your article with the aims, audience and types of article of the journal.

Remember the best journal may not be the one you read every week. It could be one read by another profession, if you are writing about multidisciplinary working, or about an issue of interest to a range of professionals or care workers.

PERSONAL DEVELOPMENT EXERCISE

As a quick check that you have picked the right journal, take a copy of their guidelines for contributors, and read down the list of instructions, ticking each one to confirm that you can deliver what they ask for in terms of word length, type of article, format, content etc. If you can't tick each item, you may have chosen the wrong target for your article.

Step 5: Approach the editor

Talk to the relevant editor or section editor as early as possible so that you get some specific guidance about what they are looking for. Your idea may be great, but if they ran something on that topic last week or month, they may not want to do it again and you may be wasting your time. (Jean Gray)

If the idea of approaching a journal editor to talk about writing an article fills you with horror, consider the advantages:

- if they are not interested, you save yourself weeks of effort writing the article only for it to be rejected
- if they are interested in the subject, but from a different angle to the one you had in mind, you have a chance to change the article plan before you write it, rather than having to rewrite it later
- they can tell you if they have already got something similar in the pipeline, have just decided to change the journal's direction, or are about to start a new section that your article would/would not fit in to – none of these things can be discovered by reading even the latest issue
- it gives you a chance to impress them and sell your idea, so that if they do express an interest, you know you already have a 'warmed up' audience for your article when it arrives
- if they are interested in your idea, you can immediately negotiate word length and deadline for delivery, so that you know what you are taking on.

Some journals are small enough to have only an editor and maybe a news reporter, so you can expect to deal directly with the editor. Larger journals will have a variety of section editors listed on their contacts page, and you can choose the one that seems most appropriate to the topic or nature of your article.

Most editors now say that they prefer to receive article ideas by email. This gives them time to look at the idea when they are not busy with other things, and you the time to prepare what you say, and polish your selling technique. However, it is still very important to prepare your idea in detail, as the editor may respond quickly wanting to know more, and won't want to wait a week while you develop your own thinking. In addition to the detailed description of the topic of your article, described above (what exactly are you going to write about? who for? for what purpose?), there are two other key questions you should answer in your initial email, before they are asked by the editor. They are:

- why now?
- why you?

The first of these is about topicality. Editors are looking for a reason for the items they feature, and you can help by giving it to them on a plate. So if you can tie your article to a particular event, date, news item, topical issue or piece of current policy, this will raise their interest in your piece. Sometimes this requires a bit of a stretch, but it is always worth a try. If you have, for example, just completed a pilot programme introducing individualised budgets for the carers of people with multiple disabilities, you could look to link your offer of an article to:

- planned fundraising activity by a charity concerned with disability
- a government announcement on action on reducing discrimination
- an awareness week about one of the disabling diseases
- the publication of a White Paper, new piece of legislation or public consultation on social care.

Bear in mind though that many journals take months to publish articles, so you need to allow for this and look far enough ahead to find a link: today's news item will be long gone by the time you write and they publish your article.

On the second question – why you? – you need to sell yourself as the author of the article. It may seem obvious if you want to write about a piece of work you have led or managed – who else could do it? But this is still an opportunity to show yourself as the kind of person who is likely to be able to write the article (knows enough about the work, can express themselves reasonably), to be reliable about delivering it (appears organised, professional and courteous), and has something extra that gives added value (interesting, we've not had an article from a social worker in our physiotherapy journal before/joint appointment between health and social care/co-written by a nurse and a carer).

So, in summary your email should tell the editor:

- what you want to write about (in detail)
- who you are aiming the article at (matching the journal's audience)
- why you are writing it (matching the kind of articles the journal publishes)
- what is going on in the world, or will happen in an appropriate timescale, that makes this article particularly relevant
- why you are the best person to write the article.

Having said all this, avoid being dogmatic about what you are offering – leave room for negotiation ('but I would be happy to discuss including the audit data, or focusing more on the patients' experience'). And keep the tone friendly and professional, not patronising – you are not offering them the chance of a lifetime for the privilege of publishing your work, just initiating a pragmatic discussion about whether you can agree on a useful article that you could write and they could publish.

> *You must be willing to work closely with editors or section editors and subeditors – and be open to having material changed where necessary. Be open to constructive criticism. While we want you to love your work, there is little room in professional publishing for authors who are over precious.* (JEAN GRAY)

All being well, after some emails and maybe a phone call, the editor (and if not the first, another from a carefully targeted journal) will express an interest, and you can move on to the next step in the process.

Step 6: Plan your article

> *Articles should be at least one of the following: informative, interesting specifically to the magazine's target audience, have something new to say, offer a fresh approach to an old subject, challenge current thought or practice, predict future trends, comment on a new development, or review current thinking.* (JEAN GRAY)

The final step before you actually start to write! This is an essential step, because few people are good enough to launch into a piece of writing, make a coherent story of it and finish with the right number of words in the right format, without doing some planning first. Planning also helps to scale down the task of writing, by reducing it to manageable pieces. Writing a 2,000 word article sounds daunting, both in terms of effort and time to be set aside: but four sections of around 400 words each, plus some introduction and a summary, is much more feasible.

This is where your researches into the journal really help you. You should have examples of articles in the same format as yours; a copy of the guidelines for contributors that tell you everything you need to know; and your email from the editor confirming what they want you to focus on, and how many words you have to do it in. With this information, you can draw up a rough article plan something like this (for an article about a project):

- introduction
- background (or issue or problem) related to the project, work, initiative, or client group
- what we did/needs to be done
- what difference it made/could be made
- lessons learned/to be taken into account
- summary.

The sections in your plan will depend entirely on the kind of article you are writing, and the guidelines from the journal, so may be different from these. The principle is that there should be a logical sequence of sections, so that the article is broken up frequently by subheadings and is easy to follow to a conclusion.

Make sure that the plan reflects what you offered the editor, and what they asked you to do; and that you have all the information you need to write the different sections – references (full citations, in the appropriate format, as per the guidelines for contributors), papers, figures, quotes or whatever. Then you are in a position to move on to writing the article, one manageable section at a time.

One tip to save you time: don't bother planning the title. In most practitioner journals, the editor will add their own title. Your witty or carefully crafted or painstakingly accurate heading is very unlikely to make it into the journal.

Step 7: Write your article

Everyone writes differently, and there is no 'right' way to do it. With the guidelines from the journal and your article plan to set the framework, it doesn't matter how you go about filling in the different sections. It is sometimes easier not to start with the introduction, but to write a more practical section first. Or you might want to write the section that requires a lot of referencing in a library, and leave the more descriptive section for an evening at home.

People also work differently when it comes to revising and finalising wording. You can go back over each section (or even paragraph) immediately, changing and improving the wording – but this can interrupt the flow and make it hard to keep the thread of what you are saying. Or you can whiz through to the end, then go back and revise later – although some people find that once they have something down, it 'sets' on the page and they find it difficult to change anything. The key things about revision are:

- make sure you do it: never write it once and send it off – there are always checks and improvements to be made
- but don't keep revising: after a couple of revisions, send it off – the subeditors will change and cut some things, and you may be asked to change things by the reviewers, so there is no point being too precious about every word.

Other useful pointers are:

- don't stop to add the full reference to the end of the article when you are in mid-flow: as long as you collected this information in full when you found the reference, it will be easy to add it later
- do a word count regularly so that you know if you are on track: otherwise you just make more work for yourself because you either have to cut and edit, or invent a new section, after you have written the article
- write in the most comfortable and speedy format for you: single spaced, double spaced, large or small font, or even by hand – and put it into the format the journal wants afterwards
- when you think it is finished, ask someone else to read it: they will spot the missing information, confusing figures or missing reference that you are too close to it to see
- spell check: by computer and by eye, since computers don't know everything!

Step 8: Pre-publication tasks

The first of these is obviously to send it in, in the format requested by the journal, and before the deadline. The journal may require both an email and a hard copy; or more than one hard copy, if they plan to send it out to reviewers. Don't forget to put the finished article into the format required: spacing, font, margins etc. Overlooking these things will only irritate the editor, and detract from the professional image you need to convey.

> *Be very respectful and aware of deadlines. We are their slaves. Time truly waits for no-one in publishing – not even the editor!* (JEAN GRAY)

If the deadline is going to be a problem, you will know this well before the date: that is the time to email the editor again and negotiate a different deadline – but only if you absolutely must. It is much better not to agree to a deadline that you may not be able to meet, and not to offer the article in the first place if you can't be sure to deliver it. The only reason for delaying a deadline should be the genuinely unpredictable emergency or crisis. Everything else – patients, clinical work, reorganisations, family demands, Christmas – are predictable, and should have been taken into account at the point at which you first discussed the article with the editor. The worst thing you can do is miss the deadline without contacting the editor; the second worst is contacting the editor just days before the deadline. They will be planning ahead on the basis of what they think you are going to deliver, and you may cause them a major problem.

Once the article is safely with the editor, there will be a pause of variable length depending on the journal, the frequency of publication and many other factors – and then you will hear from them again. Your article is unlikely to be rejected, if you have discussed it with the editor in advance, and delivered what was agreed. But you may be asked to revise it, or add to it, on the advice of the journal reviewers. Such a request is *not* a rejection: it is conditional acceptance. If you do the work as requested, then it is highly likely that the article will be published. So although nobody likes to have to go back over a piece of work and tackle it again, it is worth doing. Try to do it as soon as possible – and certainly within the timeframe suggested by the editor – and return the revised version to the editor.

If the article is to be published, you should receive a letter or email notifying you of this. You will probably also be asked to sign a form assigning copyright of the article to the journal. This is standard practice in healthcare journals, and not something usually challenged. There may also be an author's details form, requesting your title, qualifications, place of work and address for correspondence. If you have written with another person – or more – you will need to give details of the lead author. If the journal pays for articles, there may also be a form for your bank details so that payment can be made directly into your account. Needless to say, all of these should be returned promptly.

> *Give all your relevant contact details. Editors will want to contact you quickly and will expect a speedy response to messages. Do not submit an article two days before taking off on your round-the-world trip (without mobile phone). Build a reputation as a reliable author.* (JEAN GRAY)

Some journals, but not all, will send you the 'proofs' of your article to look at. Proofs show the article as it will look on the page, in columns with any boxes, pictures or figures in place. Turnaround time for correcting proofs is usually very short – it may be 24 h – and the editor (or subeditor) will usually ask for any corrections to be telephoned to them. Essential corrections, where a typo or formatting error has made the text inaccurate, are all that are expected. Examples of legitimate corrections are where numbers such as drug dosages have been changed, captions for boxes are in the wrong place, or part of a sentence has been cut, changing the meaning of the wording. This is not a chance to improve wording, or add or subtract text, since the article has been laid out on the page to fit the available space, and other features, such as boxes, pictures or adverts, have been fitted around it.

Correcting proofs, if you are asked to do so, is the final pre-publication task. If you are not sent proofs, and many journals don't do this, then the next thing you will know of your article is when it appears in the journal – so keep an eye on every issue!

After publication

Once an article has appeared, most journals send the author a copy of the relevant issue.

PORTFOLIO POINTER

Cut out any articles you have published, place them in plastic pouches and file in your portfolio. Old copies of journals or magazines don't keep well on the shelf, and are likely to be thrown out one day, so your article is safer kept elsewhere. It is also surprisingly easy, when you write more frequently, to forget what you had published where, so keeping them together makes CV writing easier. When you accumulate a moderate number of published articles, it is useful to start keeping a list of their titles, journals and summaries that you can add to, so that you don't have to start from scratch every time.

Practicalities

Some weeks after publication, notification of payment direct to your bank account, or a cheque, will follow if your journal or magazine pays its writers. If the writing was undertaken during your own time, employers don't usually expect to be given this. However, it is always a good idea to tell your employer what you are planning to write early in the process, so that if they have concerns or objections, you know about them sooner rather than later. If they want to see the draft before you send it in, you should comply with this, however irritating. It is a mistake to let them find out when someone points out your article in the latest issue.

If your article generates a letter to the journal, you may be asked to write a response. Keep this short, objective and pleasant, even if the letter writer has let rip with an assassination of your work, your views, or you personally. You will come out with much more credit than they will in the minds of other readers. *See* Chapter 26 for more about coping with the consequences of raising your head above the professional parapet.

Finally, having had one article published, it is a good idea to start immediately on the next. It gets much easier with practice, and helps to establish your name if you are seen regularly in the journals.

CHECKLIST FOR ACTION

Have you:

- decided on, and defined, what you want to write about?
- investigated a range of journals to find the best match with your article?
- contacted an editor to find someone who wants your article?

CHAPTER 18

Joining an editorial board

You never feel you're good enough – you think it's only for people of a 'higher echelon' – but you have to have the courage to have a go. (JAYNE ELTON)

There is no doubt that being on the editorial board of a professional journal is excellent experience, and is a very positive addition to a CV. But as it is generally 'by invitation only'; unlike some of the professional activities described in this book, you need an indirect rather than a direct approach to getting there. This section aims to help you refine that approach to give yourself the best possible chance of being invited to join an editorial board.

So who are these people?

The editorial board of a journal will, naturally, reflect its main aims and focus – but probably from several different perspectives, such as education, practice, research and policy. It will usually include people who are well-known names in their field, having taught, written, researched and/or practised in it. In fact, an editorial board is a microcosm of the sort of network every practitioner should be developing in order to influence the direction and quality of healthcare. This is of course another good reason for wanting to be on a board – you will gain as much from networking with fellow members as you give in support to the editor.

PERSONAL DEVELOPMENT EXERCISE

Look at the editorial boards of two different journals that you read or have access to – there is usually a list on the page that includes the staff details. How many of the names do you know? Given that these people are 'names' in your field, and closely connected to the journal you read, you should find that you recognise at least some of them. If not, think about whether you are actively building your awareness in your field: reading widely, visiting relevant websites, attending conferences if possible, or viewing conference materials online or in journals.

The functions of the board

The editor of a health- or social care-related journal is more likely to be a professional journalist than a healthcare professional. They may have edited or worked on periodicals on a wide range of topics unrelated to health. However, they will often know more about the 'big picture' of healthcare than some people who work in the NHS, because they are immersed in it every day, and have specialists on the journal staff to brief them. Still, they generally want additional input from practitioners who are health professionals and engaged in day-to-day work in the service, whether in practice, education or other sectors. Editorial boards are put together by the journal to provide advice to the editor on:

- appropriate topics and angles for articles, features and campaigns
- publisher's proposals for new sections, a new look or even a new title (*see* Box 18.1 'need to know')
- the general direction of developments in the relevant field, that should be reflected by the journal
- the quality and relevance of articles submitted to the journal
- who could be invited to contribute articles
- how the circulation, readership, profile and prestige of the journal could be increased.

BOX 18.1 Need to know: confidentiality on editorial boards

There are two main areas that editorial board members will be expected to treat as highly confidential: proposed changes to the journal, such as new sections, new layout or visuals, or a new title; and circulation figures. It is very important to comply with these expectations.

Board members are also usually expected to act as referees or reviewers for articles submitted, to find and encourage new authors, to write articles and letters, and to promote the journal generally (*see* Box 18.2 'need to know' for a cautionary word on this). All this of course happens in between meetings, and indicates the commitment required. There is real work to be done for the board – it is not simply a matter of giving 'top of the head' advice at occasional meetings.

BOX 18.2 Need to know: promoting the journal

This responsibility for promoting the journal sometimes includes an expectation that the board member will not write for other journals, or will at least give 'their' journal first refusal on article ideas. This is worth checking with the editor before accepting a place on a board, if it will prove too restrictive for your other activities.

It is worth remembering that board members are there to give advice to the editor – they don't direct him or her. The editor is ultimately answerable to the publishing company that owns the title and employs the journal staff, and this may mean that advice from the editorial board is not taken, is modified or is deferred to another month or year. So however good or exciting your ideas, or strong your feelings, be prepared to give advice and step back: the editor's decision, as they say, is final!

Getting yourself invited

Some boards seem to stay the same for a long time; others have a policy of replacing members on a rolling basis, in order to bring fresh views in and to spread the work more widely. And people move on, retire and leave for all the same reasons as they do in their day job. So there is turnover on any editorial board, and the trick is to position yourself in the editor's line of sight for a vacancy. The surest way to do so is to write regularly for the journal. Target one you are very familiar with, but consider a more specialist journal rather than one of the major, general titles. Sort out your article ideas, then talk to the editor about one of them (*see* Chapter 17 for more on writing for publication). The more professional and organised your approach to the editor, the better impression you will make. You need to follow through by delivering the article agreed: a high-quality piece of writing that matches the journal's 'guidance for contributors' and arrives before the specified deadline.

It is useful to demonstrate that you can write in a variety of styles, and that you understand the needs of the journal, by submitting letters for the letters page, and comment or opinion pieces, and offering to review books, as well as writing straightforward articles. Your aim should be to become established as a regular writer for that journal, with a reputation for good ideas, reliable delivery and sound writing skills. By dealing with the editor – or a section editor on a larger journal – by phone and email, you will also establish a personal relationship with them that will stand you in good stead.

While doing all this, you should be building up your network of contacts, and demonstrating the breadth of your knowledge and vision in articles, so that the editor can see what an asset you would be to the editorial board.

Permission and opportunity

This is also the time to ensure that you will be able to commit yourself to the board, should you be invited to join. Are you confident that your employer will release you for meetings, or that you are prepared to take leave to attend? Is your employer going to have a problem with you giving comments or writing letters to the journal? You don't need to ask the specific question in advance, since you don't know when or if an invitation will come your way. But you can find out in more general terms whether there is a complete ban on leave for professional activities, or whether other people already take time out for similar purposes.

Your own boundaries and capacity are equally important. Are you prepared to travel to the journal's headquarters? Have you got space in your home life for reading, writing and reviewing articles for the publication? It would be good to know these things before you are put in a position of having to turn down an opportunity.

PERSONAL DEVELOPMENT EXERCISE

Choose a journal whose editorial board you think you could contribute to. Now study it intensively. Look up the editorial board, and contact any members whose names you know: find a good reason to do so, such as a question about an article of theirs, or a link you have with their research or place of work. Review back issues, and note the kind of articles, features, campaigns and letters they carry. Check the list of staff, to see who is writing 'in house', and whether you could be contacting them with an article idea. Find out where the journal is physically based. Visit the publisher's website to see what else they publish. Aim to mould your professional activities to suit the journal – it will become easier the better you know the publication.

Invited to join?

If the time comes that you are invited to join the board, you will want to continue the good impression you have obviously made:

- read carefully the guidance they will send you on the role of the editorial board members and/or terms of reference of the board – this will differ between publications and between editors, so you need to know what their specific expectations are of you. If you are not going to be able to meet their expectations, because you can't attend the number of meetings required, don't have the confidence to referee articles or don't want to travel to where they will be held, then express your surprise and appreciation, but decline gracefully. It is very bad practice to accept the offer in order to have it on your CV then fail to do the work required
- prioritise the editorial board meetings – this may not be your real job, but it is a real part of the editor's job and the journal's development processes. Take it seriously and make every effort to get to meetings. Occasional crises will occur, but generally, if you have laid the groundwork with your employer and family, you should expect to go to the meetings
- get to know the other people on the board as soon as possible – look up their names, find out where they work and what they do. At your first meeting, make a point of talking to them individually. They are part of your professional network, so you may want to contact them for reasons unconnected with the work of the board. They can also give you valuable advice on the things you need to do as a board member
- when you are sent an article to review, or asked for a letter or a comment, be diligent and punctual in submitting it. Journals and journalists work to extremely tight deadlines, and if you are late submitting, or returning a phone call, they cannot wait. You hard-won reputation will suffer a severe dent if you prove unreliable and evasive.

What you can expect

Editorial board members are not usually paid, but you would expect your travel expenses to be paid for attending meetings. You will accrue all the professional and career benefits of the role, with increased profile and opportunities to network, publish and speak at related conferences. You are likely to be invited to events that the journal holds, such as award ceremonies or launches, and may be asked to judge awards it is associated with. Box 18.3 describes one nurse's experience of joining an editorial board as a result of entering her clinical work for a national award.

BOX 18.3 Joining the editorial board: one nurse's experience

Jayne Elton was invited to join the editorial board of *Practice Nurse* journal after winning the Practice Nurse of the Year award for her work on minor surgery. Here she describes the experience.

'My initial reaction was surprise – but I was absolutely chuffed, and so was my practice: it was an accolade for them. I felt as if it opened up a new experience to me, and took me outside of my own "zone". After I got over the excitement, I was anxious about going because I wasn't sure what to expect. I thought "What if I fail to deliver? I hope I'm good enough".

In reality, the board meetings were very welcoming, and very well structured in their content. They always send out an agenda first so I know what is going to be discussed. They gave me guidelines for reviewing articles.

I'm usually asked to comment on clinical issues in primary care, like prescribing, and sometimes non-clinical issues like the Knowledge and Skills Framework. What I hadn't expected was to contribute to the management of the journal as a business – thinking about how to increase sales, commenting on the layout, identifying trends that should be covered, and so on. I have really enjoyed feeling valued, and interacting with the other board members. I have been asked to contribute articles, and I still get a kick from seeing myself published.

It has had knock-on effects: I've been invited to talk at conferences and meetings, and been able to channel nurses into a course on minor surgery. A company has picked up an article I had published in *Practice Nurse* and now uses it as a teaching tool!

The challenge for me is making sure I'm earning my place by reviewing articles and writing. It's about going the extra mile. You never feel you're good enough – you think it's only for people of a "higher echelon" – but you have to have the courage to have a go.'

PORTFOLIO POINTER

When recording your place on the editorial board, also keep a record of the work you have done for the editor. A list of how many reviews you have written, and the new features ideas or campaigns that you have contributed to, is more impressive than a bald statement that 'you were there'. It is easy to forget how much work you have put in to an extracurricular role like this when refreshing your CV for a new job. And all employers know that there are, unfortunately, people who can honestly claim to have been members of great and good committees and boards, who never actually did any of the work of the group. Keep the evidence in your portfolio.

Not invited to join?

If, after all the preparation and research, you have not yet been invited to join an editorial board, it is not a wasted effort. Everything you have done helps to increase your awareness, raise your profile, hone your essential writing skills and widen your professional network. All of these developments will make you more influential in the health service, and open up a variety of other opportunities for you.

CHECKLIST FOR ACTION

Have you:

- identified a journal whose board you would like to join if asked?
- investigated it thoroughly?
- made contact with someone already on its board?
- contacted the editor with an article idea?

CHAPTER 19

Influence in meetings

Walk into every meeting assuming you have some area of skill or knowledge that no-one else there will possess. (HELEN MOULD)

Everyone knows the old jokes about meetings: they are a handy alternative to work, they are where you are when you don't want to take a phone call, a camel is a horse designed by a committee, and so on. The starker truth of the matter is that:

- meetings are meant to move things on and make things happen
- if they don't, it is the participants' fault
- it is up to you whether a meeting is useful or a waste of your time.

It is also true that it can be a very uncomfortable and embarrassing experience to be in a meeting for which you are not prepared, or when you are not clear about your role. The good news is that so many people do go unprepared to meetings, or behave badly in meetings, that it is very easy to make yourself look good and to feel in control.

This chapter is designed to ensure that you get something useful out of every meeting you go to; and that, when you have the chance to go to a meeting that will have a real influence on something you care about, you will be able to make a difference to the outcome.

The bad examples

These are so numerous, you probably know several named individuals who fall into each of the categories described below. Bad behaviour, game-playing, laziness and ineffectiveness are rife in meetings in health and social care organisations (as no doubt elsewhere) at every level, and in meetings at every point on the spectrum of significance. The same things happen in national committees, local steering groups, meetings with government ministers and professional forums. And each time, the individuals who behave badly damage their own credibility, reduce the esteem of their profession and throw away some of their precious opportunities to influence. A few examples should illustrate the depressingly common conundrum:

- *the 'too important to be here' people*: these are the ones who leave their mobiles on (and answer them without leaving the room), and spend part of the meeting time reading papers and even writing papers that are unrelated to the business in hand

- *the 'too humble to be here' people*: who don't say a word, avoid making eye contact, take industrious notes and avoid every opportunity to contribute. They often scurry away just before the end so that no-one can ask them anything
- *the 'busy busy' people*: who arrive late and make an entrance, announce that they have to leave early and can't find a date for another meeting any time in the next six months. For maximum effect, they inform the meeting that they have to go because they have a car waiting
- *the 'blissfully ignorant' people*: they haven't read the papers, or the proposals they are supposed to be commenting on, but that doesn't stop them having an opinion to share
- *the 'clever dicks'*: they take notes during the meeting on their laptop, name-drop outrageously and want to have the last word on every subject
- *the 'clowns'*: who whisper witty remarks, write notes to their neighbours, and give a performance rather than make a contribution.

> *It's not always the noisy ones that gain influence in meetings, contrary to belief, however if you don't say anything, then you never will.* (MONICA FLETCHER)

MIRROR MOMENT

Think about occasions when you have seen these behaviours in action – or even demonstrated some of them yourself. What effect did it have on the conduct of the meeting? On the business of the meeting? When others displayed these characteristics, how did you feel about that individual? However tolerant you are and however well organised the meeting, it is generally true that it takes extra effort to work in a group, and that individual behaviours that could be managed quite easily in a one-to-one encounter have a disproportionately disruptive effect in a larger group of people.

PERSONAL DEVELOPMENT EXERCISE

Next time you go to a meeting, note instances of poor meeting behaviour from others. Stop counting when you get to ten! Then practise your own meeting technique. Aim to make at least three good constructive points per meeting.

When you are invited

> *Really think about the impact you could have and don't waste it. If you are going to a meeting when the chief executive will be there, this might be your only chance to make a good first impression – don't waste it on trivial things. Think beforehand what the chief executive might be interested in hearing and write it down before saying it.* (DEB LAPTHORNE)

There are several important actions to be taken before attending a meeting that can make an enormous difference to how comfortable an experience you have, and how effective you are. Whether it is a one-off meeting, one of a series of meetings you have been to before, or the first meeting of a new group that will meet regularly, the preparatory steps are the much the same:

- *make sure you know why you have been invited*: is it you personally (your experience, expertise, reputation, skills or budget) that is wanted, or a representative from your staff group, age group, profession, organisation, region or other demographic? The vaguer the apparent reasoning ('we ought to have someone from the independent sector . . .' or 'we must have someone from nights at the meeting'), the more important it is that you put effort into the next few steps. There is nothing more frustrating than being invited as a token, with no-one having a clear idea what you're doing there when you go
- *establish what the aims of the meeting are*: to agree a statement, review a report, choose a project, decide how to achieve a target? Unless you know this – and you may have to work hard to get this information from someone – then you cannot . . .
- . . . *confirm that you are the best, right or at least an appropriate person to go*: *see* above. If they want 'someone from the independent sector', because they're discussing discharges to nursing homes, it might be that an occupational therapist, the leader of the intermediate care team, or a nursing home matron will be able to contribute more than you, if you are a home manager. This can be a particular issue if the invitation has been passed around from person to person to find 'someone who can go'. It might have been a precise and appropriate invitation to the head of community physiotherapy, but by the time it arrives with the recently-appointed sports injury specialist who has a space in his diary, it is completely inappropriate. You need to see the information that will help to decide if it should be you who attends. This will include the wording of the original invitation (especially if it was not originally sent to you); the agenda for the meeting; the list of people attending (*see* below); and if possible any minutes of a previous meeting. If you feel that you should not be attending, it is helpful to suggest a specific alternative
- *check what is expected of you*: this is an essential part of checking that it should be you who attends. Even if you were personally invited and you are not a substitute, it may be that the people inviting you have a false impression of what you can bring to the meeting. Do they expect you to speak on behalf of patients? To represent your professional peer group? To promise your department's or team's support to a project? To contribute funding? To put your name to a plan or a

statement? It can be extremely awkward to handle such misapprehensions in the middle of a meeting, if you are not able or authorised to do what is expected of you

- *know who else will be there*: at least in general terms. Knowing which organisations will be represented, whether it is an internal meeting or includes visitors, if everyone else present will be a budget holder, or part of another specific group, gives you a head-start on preparing yourself, and contributing with the right level of detail and confidentiality on the day. Again, this can be gleaned from the minutes of the previous meeting, with the list of those present, and those who sent apologies. Alternatively, if it is a new meeting with no history, see the email header, or copy list on a letter, to see who else is invited. If none of the above seems to be available, be even more cautious – you are being asked to wander blindfolded into the lion's den, carrying a tray of red meat! Contact the person who invited you and ask them to tell you who else is going – and everything else on this list, while you have their attention
- *establish what practical contribution is required from you, if you are attending*: do they want a PowerPoint® presentation, or a few words of explanation or description? Do they think you are bringing the results of a consultation, or some figures about your team's output? They may not want anything except your contribution to the discussion, but it is very scary to realise otherwise when the chair invites you to use the projector and everyone settles back to watch!

This may seem like a lot to do, for every meeting you attend, but it is definitely worth it. There are many people who seem prepared to turn up on a given date with no prior information: they must waste a lot of time and give a fairly poor impression of themselves. The time available to prepare may be short, if you are a late substitute, or simply an afterthought to the organiser. Don't take offence: take it as an opportunity to use your influence, providing it is an appropriate meeting. And get as much of this information as you can before agreeing to go.

> *Be brave: if you've been invited then you have something to say they want to hear. If you are representing a group, don't let them down by not saying something which is appropriate and relevant.* (SANDRA MELLORS)

Before the meeting

> *Good preparation is the key to influencing decisions made at meetings.* (JULIA QUICKFALL)

Having established that you have a good reason to be at the meeting, and know what is expected of you when you attend, there are a few more actions to take to prepare. You should:

- *get and read minutes of the previous meeting, if there are any*: these are a mine of information. They can tell you not only what happened, but who was there, who was invited but didn't go, what actions should have taken place before this meeting, why they decided to invite a new person, what sort of issues they discussed and at what level, how formal the meeting is, how often the group meets, and many other things

- *get and read the agenda and papers for this meeting*: many people do this at the last minute, but this leaves you no time to find additional information, consult others or prepare your own thoughts. Try to read them no later than the day before – this may be when you find out that they are expecting you to make a presentation, or that the chief executive will be there. Give yourself a chance to prepare
- *gather background information or reference material*: you don't need to do an entire literature search, but having a relevant project report, set of figures, name of a useful contact or description of a similar project elsewhere to hand could give you something useful to contribute in the meeting. Reading the background policy paper, or local protocol, can prevent you putting your foot in it by displaying ignorance about something that everyone else is familiar with
- *confirm that you will be attending*: as a matter of courtesy and efficiency. If you absolutely must arrive late or leave early (for a very, very good reason), let the organiser know so that, if you are needed for a particular item or decision, you don't wreck the meeting by missing it
- *check what you are authorised to say, agree or promise with the appropriate person or people*: so that you are ready to meet the expectations the meeting has of you. If they think you are going to commit your team to try a new way of working, or represent the views of your staff group on a national committee, you should not go the meeting only to say 'I'll have to check that out and get back to you'. Needless to say, if you are not empowered to do anything in the meeting, it is likely that you shouldn't be there
- *prepare any paper or information that you have been asked to bring in support of an agenda item in good time*, and send it to the secretary well before the meeting (*see* Chapter 24 on writing papers for meetings). It is very annoying for meeting attendees to receive papers piecemeal because they were submitted late. Ideally, you should never 'table' a paper – unless it is so short and clear that you could have managed without a paper, it is unfair to expect participants to read it on the spot and make any sensible comment on it. It takes extra time out of the meeting, annoys everyone, and at worst suggests that you are not only inefficient, but may be trying to hide something
- *if you are going to speak* to a particular agenda item but haven't been asked to do a paper, *consider whether it would be useful to do so*. It will be reassuring to you to know that, even if you get muddled or rushed on the day, people will be able to refer to your paper for the full picture. As meetings sometimes run out of time and rush items, it may be very important that this option is available. If you are going to do this, let the chair or secretary know, so that your paper can be distributed with the rest.

Meeting basics

Know how to behave in a formal meeting (addressing the meeting through the chair); sometimes it is worth 'keeping your powder dry' – letting others make a point and listening, then making the point you wish to near the end of the discussion: that often gets you what you want. (Joanna Parker)

Walking into a meeting room can be a nerve-wracking experience, even if you know the group and have been there before. Many of us don't feel at our best in larger groups of people, and the unpredictable behaviour that is so common at meetings means that even more confident people can feel 'wrong-footed' and embarrassed. So taking some control of the situation, and minimising the anxiety potential of factors that are under your control, is helpful. For example, such simple measures as making sure you arrive in good time, and don't have to rush in late, hot and bothered, are a good start. So make sure you know where the meeting room or venue is, and don't rely too much on public transport timetables. Other good moves are to introduce yourself to people either side of you, turn your mobile phone off, and talk to people rather than burying yourself in your papers. To reduce the number of strangers you will be speaking in front of, make a point of introducing yourself to some of them before the meeting starts, and make a note of their names and where they are from.

If you may have a difficult situation or new idea, lobby members of the meeting group prior to the meeting – at least you will know what you are dealing with and you might get people on side. (Barbara Stuttle)

Introductions

Listening is a key tactic. If items on the agenda are boring or irrelevant, use the time to 'people watch' and work out the motivation and style of colleagues. It will really help when you try to persuade them of something later. (Helen Mould)

When the meeting starts, and people round the table are invited to introduce themselves, it is very useful to make a note of their names and where they are from or who they are representing, in a way that shows where they are sitting in relation to you (*see* Figure 19.1). This allows you to refer to them by name later ('as Jim said') which is polite; to address your comments to the right individuals round the table ('could our primary care colleagues tell us more about . . .?') which is impressive; and to speak to them after the meeting or later, if you think they may be a useful contact. Once you have left the meeting it is easy to forget who 'that man from social services who is developing the business plan' is. And there are generally far too many people at any meeting for you to remember anything about them by the time the round table introductions have concluded.

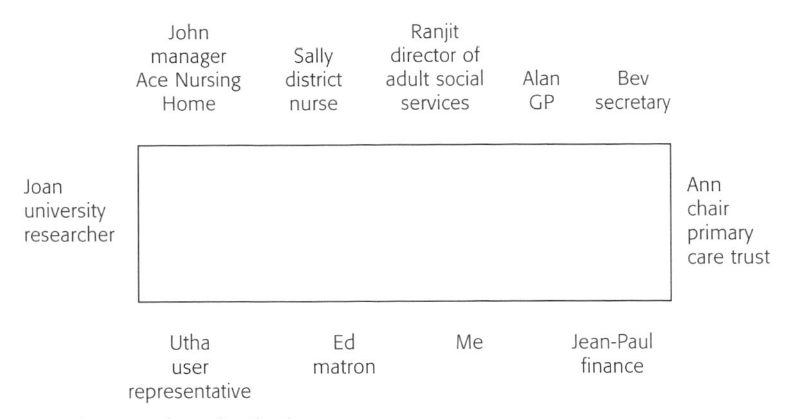

Figure 19.1 Meeting attenders: sketch plan

> *The tea and chat in the middle of a meeting can be more important than the agenda. Being remembered for who you are lasts a lot longer than what you said.* (Helen Mould)

Introducing yourself

This can be a nightmare moment if you are shy or feeling intimidated by the other attendees at the meeting. Conversely, if you are very comfortable and familiar with the group, it can seem like a boring bit of business to be got through as swiftly as possible. In either case it is easy to waste a very good opportunity to make an impression on relevant people. (Remember, if they have no relevance to you, your work or your areas of interest, you probably shouldn't be in the meeting in the first place!) How many times have you heard people, when invited to introduce themselves:

- mutter inaudibly
- gabble incomprehensively
- bark aggressively
- say 'I think everyone knows me' airily.

When it is your turn to introduce yourself, take a deep breath and smile. This relaxes your throat, warms up your tone and makes you appear friendly and confident. Then say your name clearly, and consciously slow down a little from your normal speaking pace – it won't sound slow to others, just clear. Look round the table and meet people's eyes. If the chair has invited you to do so – or if it seems important – also say where you are from, and why you are there.

As well as making a good impression on others, this also helps you in two ways:

- by acting confident and relaxed, you will inevitably feel a bit more so
- by making an effective early contribution, you have 'broken your duck', and will find it easier to enter the discussion with other comments or information later.

PERSONAL DEVELOPMENT EXERCISE

Practise your personal introduction outside of meetings as well as in meetings. If this is a nightmare moment for you, practise alone until it feels more comfortable. Work out what form of your name you want to give – do you feel embarrassed being 'Gilly', 'Rosie' or 'Johnny' in meetings? How will you describe your job and organisation in the easiest and most meaningful terms? Some NHS trusts have lengthy and unwieldy names that could be shortened. Some job titles are frankly weird and could be better expressed by saying what you lead on, or are responsible for. Then look your mirror, partner, best friend or colleagues in the eye, and deliver a clear and concise introduction. If you are very confident in introducing yourself, still practise. You may have lapsed into the habit of gabbling, or dropping your voice at the end of your name because you think everyone knows you anyway. Slow down, smile, and deliver it with conviction.

Making a contribution in the meeting

Prepare your pitch and provide evidence and data – have a strategy or plan. (Fran Woodard)

The point of being at a meeting is almost invariably to contribute something. Occasionally you might be there only to listen – but usually only if it has been clearly stated that you have 'observer status' (*see* Box 19.1), and either you or the chair makes this clear at the start. Otherwise, your fellow participants will be expecting you to say something constructive at some point. The exception to this rule may be the very large committee, where the items on the agenda at one meeting may be relevant to other members but not to you, and so lead to a discussion to which you cannot contribute. If this is the case in more than one meeting, however, you (and the chair) should probably question why you are a member.

BOX 19.1 Observer status in meetings

When a person has formal observer status, in a formal meeting, they are usually placed away from the main meeting table, or at one end, and not expected to contribute. Observer status is given as a courtesy gesture, for example to officials from devolved administrations in a meeting concerning health services in England. The chair may invite observers to speak, or they may ask to do so, but they do not usually contribute without this courtesy first.

In a less formal meeting, observers may be people who are not formal members of the group that is meeting, and so are not able to vote on an issue, or have their views taken into account in decisions, but who are welcome to contribute comments. The chair should make this clear at the beginning of the meeting.

Offering to take notes can be really helpful, especially when you are less confident. It forces you to listen and understand. It gives you 'permission' to ask for clarification and your 'take' as an argument may well stand. (Helen Mould)

So, how do you make a constructive contribution?

If you believe in something, say it and make sure you are heard. Sometimes it's like a seed – you say something, then add bits of information and see the ideas grow as people grasp what you mean. (Barbara Stuttle)

First, obey the rules of conduct. In a very formal committee, members will have been told how to contribute at the beginning of the meeting, or will know from previous meetings. If nothing has been said, observe how others do it when introducing themselves or making early contributions. This may mean raising a hand, finger or pen first to catch the chair's eye, then waiting to be invited by name. You may have to turn on a microphone in front of you, or wait for someone to bring you one. In a meeting this formal, it is usual to address all comments to the chair, rather than speaking directly to other members. The chair will then invite the other person to respond, if this is appropriate. Because these procedures can be slow and cumbersome, it is even more important to make your contribution brief, clear and to the point. Note how members are referred to: a meeting like this may be one of the last remaining places where members are called 'Mr', 'Mrs' or 'Professor'. Whatever others do in this respect, you should do too, no matter how odd it feels. To influence, you have to play the game by the rules. Rudeness, bad behaviour or non-conformity gives people an excuse to ignore your view and downgrade your credibility.

Few meetings are this formal, but vestiges of this way of conducting meetings remain in lots of other forums: assessing exactly how much formality is required in your meeting is the trick to master. Taking notice of the chair's cues before and while joining the discussion is the least you should do. If in doubt, err on the side of formality rather than informality.

Reflecting too much means you don't say anything and so are overlooked in meetings – people don't recognise you are there. Speaking too soon means you are seen to be interrupting and a nuisance. (Judith Whittam)

It is always useful to jot down a word or two about your point or idea while waiting to speak: this gives you confidence that you won't forget it as soon as you have the attention of the meeting, and allows you to shape it into a more coherent form.

Although some emotion is required to enable people to understand your point of view and come on board, if you are too emotional you will lose the clarity of the argument. (Julia Quickfall)

Use your facts, examples and background material to give weight to your point.

Saying 'the district nurses won't like it' may be true, but is easier to dismiss than '60% of the district nurses who did our survey were opposed to closing the AB centre' or 'closing the CD centre last year led to a 10% rise in district nurse turnover' (or travel costs, or whatever).

> *Don't win the battle but lose the war – don't be frightened to play the long game.* (Alison Norman)

Acknowledge others' points positively when responding, even if you totally disagree with them. It is possible to do this without appearing to endorse them – which you may want to avoid. For example, if the estates manager says 'Well, the district nurses will have to lump it, they're always complaining about something', your reply 'I realise there are reasons why this has to happen, but I think we should look objectively at the DNs' concerns' acknowledges his comment without agreeing with it.

The response 'I know, but I think we should look objectively at the DNs' concerns', however, gives the impression that you agree that the district nurses are a pain.

A confrontational response – 'That's no way to talk about them' – is generally not appropriate in the meeting: everyone else will be aware of the rudeness, and it doesn't need to be pointed out. Let people condemn themselves out of their own mouths. The exception to this is comments that cannot be allowed to pass unchallenged, such as discriminatory remarks, or personal abuse. If these occur, it is the chair's responsibility to deal with them.

> *Fact-based information given in meetings can enhance the profile and influence you have. But don't steam-roller others – listen to their opinions too.* (Kay East)

The most important characteristic of a constructive contribution to a meeting is that it moves things on. Ideally (so, in real life, not very often), every comment or contribution should add something new, move the discussion forward, and lead towards the achievement of the aims of the meeting. So, when you speak, try to:

- bring in a new idea
- offer a relevant fact or example
- raise a question that will make people think
- summarise key points from the discussion in preparation for the next step
- suggest a new angle to the issue which will help to clarify it.

What you should not do is:

- speak for the sake of saying something
- repeat the previous point in different words
- speak for too long because you have the attention
- make a pre-prepared statement on behalf of your organisation or team where it isn't directly relevant to the discussion

- be rude or sarcastic, or interrupt others' contributions
- constantly reference your own work to demonstrate how good it is.

> *Always take time to encourage and support less confident colleagues. If a shy person makes a comment, say something like 'I really agree' or 'Well put.'*
> (HELEN MOULD)

Non-constructive contributions from others

If unhelpful, rambling or downright rude comments are made in general by others in the meeting, it is the chair's problem. However it may happen that they are directed at you, or that someone seems intent on arguing a point with you. The key is to stay calm and objective, addressing the point, not the emotion or underlying message. Remember, the better you behave, the more the other person puts themselves in the wrong. Saying to the person, in a tone of finality, 'I've noted what you say', or 'It seems we are not going to agree on this', may help to call a halt without you having to concede any points with which you disagree.

> *Notice where influence would be more effective outside of the meeting.*
> (SUZANNE HILTON)

Of course, the chair should intervene to stop a discussion turning into a personal argument at an early stage. If this doesn't happen, and it goes on longer than you are comfortable with, you can always turn to the chair and prompt their help by saying 'Would you like us to continue this discussion another time?'

Action points

During the meeting, it is a good idea to note down any actions you are asked, or offer, to undertake. Sometimes minutes of a meeting are not written up for weeks, and not distributed until shortly before the next meeting. If you leave it too late, you may be put in the embarrassing position of having to admit that you have not done what you said you would. Make your notes sufficiently detailed that they will make sense the next day or week after the meeting. Scribbling 'survey' or 'website' next to the agenda item may not trigger the memory that you offered to send a copy of the full results of the district nurse survey to the secretary to send out with the minutes, or that you were asked to ensure that your organisation's latest briefing paper is downloadable from the website. Using the agenda paper for both the diagram of who is present (*see* Figure 19.1) and your list of actions means that you have them linked to the right meeting, with the date and agenda items to remind you of the context.

After the meeting

When it's all over it generally isn't over. Try not to rush away. As the meeting breaks up is the time to consolidate the good impression you have made with important contacts. Take advantage of the relaxation after the formal part of the meeting to have a word with specific people and give them your contact details if you think contact between meetings would be useful. Say goodbye to the chair if you have the chance.

Then, of course, make sure you deliver those actions you promised to undertake. When the minutes arrive, never file them unread until next time. Check that they record your views accurately, if ascribed (if not, you or someone will need to ask for this to be corrected at the next meeting) and that you haven't missed any actions. Note the date and place of the next meeting.

Finally, observe the rules agreed at the meeting regarding confidentiality of discussions and papers when responding to questions from others, or telling them about the meeting (*see* 'need to know' Box 19.2). If you do share information that was given in confidence in the meeting, verbally or by sharing papers, you can be sure that someone will find out. And at the very least, you will not be invited back, and so lose your opportunity to influence. Depending on the importance of the information 'leaked' in this way, more serious action could follow.

BOX 19.2 Need to know: The Chatham House Rule

You may hear the expression 'Chatham House rules' used at a meeting. This phrase originated in 1927 with the Royal Institute of International Affairs, based in Chatham House in London. The Institute is a membership organisation that analyses international issues. The Rule (there is only one) was refined in 1997 and 2002. It states that: 'When a meeting, or part thereof, is held under the Chatham House Rule, participants are free to use the information received, but neither the identity nor the affiliation of the speaker(s), nor that of any other participant, may be revealed'. Its aim is to encourage openness and sharing of information by allowing anonymity to the speakers. It also allows people to give their own views as opposed to those of their organisation. *See* www.chathamhouse.org.uk/index.php?id=14.

Using the Chatham House Rule is of course different from saying that nothing said or heard in the meeting can be repeated outside; if this degree of confidentiality is required, it must be respected absolutely. If in doubt, check with the chair.

KEY POINTS TO REMEMBER

- Any meeting is only as useful as you make it – if you go to boring meetings that you have nothing to contribute to, do something about it.
- Good meeting behaviour creates a good impression that enhances your credibility and influence – even if you don't have anything earth-shattering to say.

Chairing a meeting

Even small groups or team meetings provide a good place to practise 'chairing' a meeting – even if it isn't called that. The overall aim of the chair is to encourage the good behaviours listed above, and discourage the bad, in order to get the business of the meeting done in the time allowed. To do this, it helps to:

- set a good example: with friendliness, speaking to everyone beforehand, switching off your phone, making eye contact with everyone in the meeting, and listening to all contributions
- be organised: make sure you have all the papers, pens and equipment that you need
- tell everyone clearly about the 'ground rules' at the start of the meeting
- gently steer people away from bad habits and behaviours – don't let them get away with it.

Most of all, watch and learn from people who are good at chairing the meetings you attend. It is a real skill, and role models are the most valuable teachers.

CHECKLIST FOR ACTION

Have you:

- practised introducing yourself with confidence and poise?
- tried out good meeting technique and made constructive contributions at recent meetings?
- identified someone who is a good meeting chair to learn from?

CHAPTER 20

The use and abuse of groups

> *Groups are like families, you don't have to like everyone in the group but you have to find a way to make it work to get the task done.* (DEB LAPTHORNE)

Most of us, in our professional lives at least, like to be asked to join a group. Even if, as a child, we shunned the Brownies and preferred Solitaire to team games, in our professional lives being invited to join a group feels like a compliment. Being asked to join a regional forum or national committee, or a group of experts in our field, is a real thrill the first time it happens – even if we try to be nonchalant about it. And however effective we are at individual activities such as letter writing, there is no doubt that people working together in a group can have more influence.

So groups are a really good opportunity to influence change and development. And they can also undoubtedly be good for your career, if you perform well in them. Many people with senior positions in national organisations, and many of the most senior and well-known clinicians, learned their influencing and leadership skills initially through work in local groups. A CV that demonstrates that you have done your own job very well in a variety of posts illustrates only that. But a career that combines developing expertise in your own job with the breadth of contribution to wider work – through membership of groups – is much more impressive. It indicates that you have more to offer, you know how to work with others outside of your immediate team, you have initiative and commitment, you are organised enough to manage both at once – and so on.

It is tempting to want to start at the top with a place at the table on a national committee or steering group. But this is unlikely to happen. No-one is going to risk inviting you to join such a group without some evidence that you are reasonably well informed about the key subjects (which is why developing your awareness is so important), and that you are able to contribute effectively. There are experts, enthusiasts and committed people throughout health and social care who are not good at making a point, sharing their resources, or operating well in groups. To demonstrate that you are not one of these, and to make yourself a likely candidate for the seriously influential groups, you need a track record and a profile. Becoming a member of other groups is the way to start building these, and to begin to use your influencing skills.

Don't worry about how members of local or specialist groups can possibly appear on the radar of professional leaders or national group members: health and social care is a remarkably small world, with very well-developed informal networks. Names become known, people are always asking for good contacts, and other people are very good at sharing their networks and spreading the opportunities around. The fact that so many frontline clinicians and managers already sit on key groups means that there is a direct line into the service through which new 'stars' can be spotted.

Types of group with potential to influence

There is a wide range of groups you can join that will provide valuable opportunities to develop your network and your influencing skills.

Local professional forums and special interest groups can both influence local practice, and make representations at national level too. They are helpful for keeping up to date with developments in your field, and local work builds a series of achievements and outcomes that you can cite in your CV, and when networking with contacts. Contributing as a forum to national consultations (*see* Chapter 23 on writing letters) is an ideal way to get your group's name known, and, attached to a thoughtful, informed, constructive set of comments, it enhances the reputation of everyone in the group.

Project groups are time-limited groups, focused on delivering a specific piece of work. But as well as enabling you to influence the project in hand, they provide a chance to meet new contacts from outside your organisation or department, and to learn something from the process about unfamiliar subjects (such as budgeting, health and safety legislation or project management) that you can use elsewhere.

Network groups tend to be large groups, scattered geographically and more often linked by email and newsletters than meetings. It is easy to be a passive member of this kind of group, receiving information but never contributing anything. But conversely, being active and engaged in a network is a very easy way to build a good reputation and get yourself noticed. If you are one of the few who does respond to circulated questions, acknowledges receipt of newsletters and makes suggestions for developing the network, it will be noted and remembered.

Journal clubs/research groups are often focused on learning and development, but there is no reason why they should not lead to more external activity too. Influencing the adoption of good practice from elsewhere, or the implementation of valid research findings locally, are tangible outcomes from the work of a group like this that demonstrate members' initiative and commitment.

Union or professional organisation committees are usually populated by people who have been through a clearly defined process that may involve local and regional structures and election procedures. They offer fewer opportunities for people to become members simply by volunteering. Given this, the expectation on members is all the greater, and it is even more important that members work effectively and professionally. Bad behaviour such as missing a lot of meetings or failing to represent the mandated views tends to come out embarrassingly in the professional journals.

The effort of going through election procedures is usually well repaid by the training given and experience obtained from work for these organisations.

National advisory, reference or steering groups are genuinely influential, often contributing significantly to the direction of policy, service or practice development. They also provide the best opportunity to enhance not only your individual reputation, but that of the professional group you come from. When someone says 'that therapist was really good in that meeting', all therapists get a little bit of the credit. Conversely, if someone has to say 'the pharmacist obviously didn't know anything about electronic transfer of prescriptions', then the suspicion lurks that all pharmacists are similarly ill-informed. There are still astonishing degrees of separation between different professions in the NHS, and between health and social care, and a mutual lack of comprehension between professionals in these fields and other groups such as civil servants, so massive over-generalisations tend to take the place of intelligent thought. The best way to turn this to advantage is to epitomise the efficient, informed, constructive practitioner or manager, and let the rest of your profession reap the benefit.

MIRROR MOMENT

Think about any groups you belong to. Are you an active member, or a passive one – or so passive as to be a lapsed member? Consider what you get out of membership of the group, and what you bring to the group. Try to score each group for its usefulness to you (1 = not useful at all, don't know why I go, 5 = very useful, highlight of my job) and your usefulness to it (1 = they wouldn't notice if I wasn't there, 5 = the group would fold if I didn't go). Decide what action you ought to take based on these scores. If you don't belong to any group at all, think about why. Never invited? Don't like groups? No time? You will need to address these issues if you are to extend your influence.

Using groups constructively

> *Purpose and timescale are the key to making the most of groups and technology means they can, where suitable, be virtual. Bringing people together is expensive time lost to 'day jobs', travel and administration. The benefits need to outweigh the costs – actual and hidden.* (Sue Norman)

As with bad behaviour in meetings discussed in the last chapter, examples of misuse of groups are legion. Before looking at constructive membership, let's get some of the biggest faults out of the way:

- *joining but not attending*: I have known groups that met for over a year with some members never attending a single meeting

- *'collecting' groups*: some people say yes to every group, and cannot sustain attendance or contribution to most of them. It is better to belong to fewer and be a well-regarded member
- *CV padding*: related to the above, people say yes to every group, fail to attend or contribute, but list the group membership on their CV because it looks impressive. Remember, health and social care is small world. People notice and remember
- *prioritising individual benefit over group aims*: helping the group to achieve its aims will reflect well on you, but some members disregard this and are only prepared to do things that directly benefit them
- *failing to deliver actions between meetings*: just turning up is not enough. This is lazy membership, and will not gain you any credit
- *undermining the work of the group in other settings*: if you are going to have a conflict of interest, you should not join the group. But being party to the group's work and decisions, then rubbishing them outside of the meetings, is highly unprofessional.

Having chosen or been invited to join an appropriate group – one that shares your aims and interests, and will build your networks and influence – it is worth putting some positive effort into it.

> *If you want a group to do something for you, be honest and clear about what you are expecting and what you will give in return.* (BARBARA STUTTLE)

Before your first meeting, check it out as described in the previous chapter about meetings generally, so that you know why you have been asked (or volunteered), what is expected of you, and what authority you have to represent views or commit your resources. Arm yourself with useful facts, figures, background documents and history. Check on the use of substitutes (*see* Box 20.1)

BOX 20.1 Use of substitutes in a group

Some groups have strict rules about not sending a substitute if the original member cannot attend. If they are not made explicit, check before delegating your place, to avoid putting someone else in an invidious position at the meeting.

If you can, and must, send a substitute:

- give them the same background information that you have
- brief them about the nature of the meeting
- agree what sort of contribution they will make (are they going to contribute to the discussion but not take decisions, or act as if they were you and do anything you would have done?)
- check with them soon afterwards to hear about the meeting, and pick up any actions to be taken before the next meeting.

Don't:

- send them with inadequate information
- restrict them to a listening brief (unfair to them and the group)
- make them a permanent substitute: if you don't intend to go again, get them accepted as a member in their own right.

Above all, don't sabotage them with poor preparation in order to make yourself look good: I have known it happen! If there is any danger that they will outshine you at the meeting, this should spur you on to improve your own meeting performance.

> *Take time to get to know members of the group – their strengths, talents and areas of expertise.* (SUE BORAN)

Once you have joined the group, get to know the other members by talking to them before and after meetings, noting their names, organisations and positions, and any special interests they have. Contact some between meetings, where you have something specific to ask or offer, and make them part of your network. Look out for other opportunities to work with them: you could ask one to review a draft of an article, or send them a piece of research they might be interested in.

In the group meetings, make sure your contributions help move the discussion forward, and that your background information, facts and figures are useful to the group (*see* Chapter 19, Influence in meetings). Volunteer to take on actions between meetings, checking facts, finding references or contacts or drafting something. Then, of course, make sure you deliver what you said you would, and not the day before the next meeting! Help the group by offering to host a meeting, if you are in a position to do so, or to lead a subgroup, or distribute notes. Many groups with great potential flounder and finish because all the work of the group falls onto a few people – it should be spread around, and every member should expect to do some of the more tedious tasks.

Being honest

There can be moments in a group when you are asked for your opinion or for information, and you suddenly realise that you are the only person there speaking about your profession or area of work, your peers' point of view or your organisation. Your input is being sought and, if you have built credibility and respect through your contributions and approach to the group, what you say will be taken at face value. It will form part of the picture that will influence the value judgements, policy development or decisions made by the group. The gratification this gives – after all, you wanted influence, didn't you? – is often tempered, in any sensible person, by a sudden sense of responsibility. You want to be sure that your contribution warrants this degree of serious attention, and that the impetus it gives to decision making is in the right direction.

There are three simple tests to apply to anything you contribute, it should be:

- informed
- impartial
- honest.

You cannot know everything about your subject, but there is no excuse for speaking on the basis of ignorance of easily available and essential background information. If you are on a project group, you must know all about the project, its history, rationale, aims and progress. If you are on a policy group, you should have read the relevant policy documents and know about current consultations or recent White Papers. Network contacts are very useful for giving a wider perspective and alternative models that can be drawn upon to provide different examples and options for the group. Only if you are speaking from a position of knowledge and information can your contribution be trusted.

Whatever the subject, you should also have read about or discussed it enough to know the pros and cons of the arguments, and to understand perspectives and experiences other than your own. One common problem in groups is people who can talk a lot about their own work, unit or example, but appear unable to apply the learning from that experience to an objective discussion of a broader topic. So their contribution is stuck at the level of 'In Manchester, we do it this way . . .', when what is important to the group is to consider the relative merits of different ways of introducing a new initiative.

Objectivity is important. Your purpose in the group is not to ensure that the decision is to do things your way, or to endorse your point of view. It is to harness the collective knowledge and intelligence of the group to find the best way to achieve the group's aims. A good example of this is in groups planning the implementation of policy – whether setting up new services, extending non-medical prescribing or introducing new hybrid professional roles. As a professional invited to join such as group, your role is not to ensure that your particular profession gets what it wants from the policy, or that your own view of what 'should' be done carries the day. Your role, with the rest of the group, is to make sure that the services, prescribing or new roles are as good and useful to patients as they can possibly be. It is like being with a group of people in a minibus going to London – you are not expected to grab the wheel and make them go to Margate instead because you think the sea air is healthier. You are there to help steer a smooth, safe route to the capital in the shortest possible time.

The honesty of your contribution depends a lot on how you present it. It is easy to find yourself talking in generalities, and if people don't question them, decisions can be swayed by information that has not been challenged for accuracy or relevance. It is helpful to say where your information comes from, and good background work will give you plenty of material. It might be easy to say 'nurse practitioners are as good as doctors at diagnosing minor illness', but it would be more impressive and more truthful to mention the randomised controlled trials that have shown this – and to mention that the nurses' consultations in these trials took longer than the doctors'. But what if you don't have research evidence to hand for every statement – which will usually be the case? Then you can indicate the basis for your statement with useful phrases like:

- 'In my experience . . .' ('. . . as nurse practitioners become more experienced their consultation time matches that of GPs')
- 'In my practice [we do things this way] . . . but I know there are practices where [they do something else]'
- 'There is a pilot study going on in Sunderland where . . . and I can get more information from the person leading the project'
- 'My understanding is that . . . but I'll check that in the literature/with my professional organisation/at our next regional meeting'.

Then, if your contribution is allowed to guide decision making, everyone will know the basis for it, and you will know that you have acted honestly in influencing the outcome.

What you should avoid doing, when invited to contribute in a situation where you are the only person able to speak about a subject, is, of course:

- twisting the facts to suit your view, because no-one knows enough to contradict you
- guessing, because you don't want to look ill informed
- exaggerating, to give weight to your point.

If your input to the group passes the triple test of being honest, objective and informed, you should feel confident that you have acted in good faith and with professional integrity. Since professionals operate under codes of conduct that cover all of their activities, not just their clinical practice, this is essential. No-one can predict the outcome of any project, policy or initiative, and sometimes things will go wrong. It is helpful to be clear in your own mind that your contribution to the collective decision making that influenced the work was justified and given in good faith.

Setting up your own group

Instead of – or as well as – joining other groups, you could set up your own. This is invariably a lot more work and effort than contributing well to another group, and you still need to ensure that your contributions to your own group are worthwhile and effective – so setting up a group is not something to be undertaken lightly. Only do so if there is no effective alternative, then consider these guidelines to make the group work for you:

Purpose

Be very clear what the purpose of the group is. Ideally it should be describable in a sentence: 'to co-ordinate the therapists' response to the consultation on registration', or 'to manage the introduction of clinical supervision into the unit'. The aim can be developed collectively into terms of reference later, if the group needs them.

Timescale

> *Only keep a group together for the lifetime of its need and don't be afraid to change membership as the outcomes change.* (JUDITH WHITTAM)

It is a good idea to have a time limit on a new group, partly so that group members know what they are signing up for, and also because it focuses minds on achieving the aims. A group set up to 'provide support to therapist prescribers' could be kept busy for years without ever feeling it has achieved its aim. A group set up for nine months would focus much more closely on identifying and supporting the first cohorts of therapists to emerge from training, learning what they need to help them translate their education into practice, and making sure that someone plans to provide it.

Functioning

A group does not necessarily have to meet face-to-face, although many groups that set out to work at a distance find that they need to meet occasionally. There is a dynamism to discussion with people in the room that is hard to reproduce through email, chat rooms or by other electronic means (*see* below for more about teleconferencing, videoconferencing and online meetings). However, these methods can be very effective for elements of the work, and a combination of approaches might be the best solution. It is a good idea to let prospective members know what combination of methods is likely to be used and what the frequency of each method will be, as this will affect their ability to join.

Members

Try to recruit some people who you know are knowledgeable, keen and good contributors, even if the group is open to others too. Otherwise you may be unlucky and get a group full of people who sit back and wait to be informed.

Sharing responsibilities

As the founder of the group, you may feel a responsibility to take on all the onerous tasks initially. It is good to share these amongst group members as soon as possible. This both saves you from overload, and makes others feel ownership of, and commitment to, the group. If you continue to organise the meetings, take the notes, provide the venue and carry out the actions, others will soon feel that the whole business is your enterprise, and they are not needed.

Funding

If there is no formal funding for the group, sharing the hosting of face-to-face meetings, or other forms of contribution in kind, becomes even more important to ensure that one organisation or individual does not invest disproportionately in the group. If money is involved, it either needs to be handled through the host organisation, via a separate budget line that you can monitor, or, if you take contributions from members of the group, you will need to have a separate account (usually with two signatories), and a treasurer with responsibility for it. This should be covered in your terms of reference.

Planning the work

Some form of project plan for the work the group needs to do to achieve its aim, with some milestones, helps keep the group focused. Achieving each milestone is encouraging, and provides some tangible demonstration that the group is working, which encourages existing members, and will help to recruit new ones to replace the inevitable leavers.

Growing the group

Welcoming new members warmly, ensuring that they are introduced to others and brought up to speed on actions to date, is important. Involving them in actions and tasks early on helps to cement their engagement. Groups can easily divide into cliques, or even split, if there is seen to be a gulf between the original members and those who joined later.

Business and social aspects

A social element to the group, such as sharing a meal, may be important to build trust and commitment in a group, particularly if it is under pressure, tackling a very difficult or demanding task, or suffering criticism. It is usually wise to keep the business and social elements of a meeting or occasion separate, especially with regard to funding of the social element. This ensures that the group can't be accused of either losing sight of its business aims, or misusing its funding: both of which tend to alienate some members, and, more importantly, funders.

Successes and achievements

These are always worth acknowledging and celebrating in some way, to reward group members for their work and spur on efforts towards the next goals. When a group is in addition to someone's daily work, they deserve acknowledgement of the extra work they have put in – and shared celebrations always help to build the cohesion of the group. For new groups, even relatively minor early milestones are worth marking, since they represent not only achievements on the way to the bigger aims, but milestones in the life of the group.

Departing members

Whether your group achieves all its aims and disbands, or members leave one at a time through natural turnover, it is a good idea to write to departing members to thank them for their contribution. You may want to keep them in your network, or call on them again in future, and a 'good ending' to their involvement in the group will leave a positive impression and build your credit with them. If you can include reference in the letter to any specific element of the work that the individual undertook ('we are especially grateful to you for taking on the editing of the good practice booklet . . .') , or to the nature of their general contribution ('your knowledge of information systems was invaluable . . .') to personalise it, this is even better. Reference to the dates during which they were a member and the full title of the group is helpful. This will remind the individual of what it was all about when they look at the letter years later (*see* portfolio pointer below); and, for the group, a copy in the file acts as a record of who was involved and what skills were in the group at different times.

PORTFOLIO POINTER

If you receive such a letter when you leave a group, file it in your professional portfolio. It is surprising how things fade from the memory during a busy working life. When you are next updating your CV and looking for relevant experience to include, it is useful to be able to look back and find details of what you did, when and to what end in which group. Remember that employers, educational institutions or awarding bodies are as interested in activities that demonstrate your commitment and capabilities in practical ways as they are in your formal qualifications or list of previous posts. If you don't receive a letter of thanks when you leave a group, take time to write a summary of the group, its aims and achievements, as well as the dates you were a member and any specific contribution you made. File this in your portfolio for future reference.

Alternatives to face-to-face group meetings

Teleconferencing

This can work very well, even with a large number of participants, if it is properly managed. Although there is a cost, it is still likely to be cheaper than the travel and time-out costs of a face-to-face meeting, and the benefits of freeing people from the time and stress of travel are considerable. Teleconferencing probably works best when:

- there are fewer than eight participants
- the participants know each other
- the meeting is structured, with an agenda and all papers sent out in advance
- items to be discussed are practical and familiar to participants
- the meeting is expected to take no longer than an hour and a half at most.

Meetings with other characteristics can also work, but are harder to manage.

There are two types of teleconference – those moderated by a meeting facilitator from the company supplying the facility, or shared calls where all participants dial in, but no-one from the company is on the line.

Moderated calls

These are useful for larger meetings, because the moderator (or host) can ensure that only one person can be heard at a time, and can see from their equipment when someone wants to come in with a comment. They co-ordinate introductions and speakers, and manage the technical aspects of multiple callers. These conferences are easy for participants, who are sent joining instructions (a number to dial and a code to insert when prompted) then are guided through the whole process by the moderator.

No external moderator

Teleconferencing with no external moderator is better for smaller groups. For these calls, members are given a number to dial and a code number to insert. When they enter the code, they are usually asked to say their name. This is recorded automatically, and, when the conference opens, the recording will be played back announcing '"So and so" has joined the meeting'. If they are cut off for any reason, other members will be informed when they are interrupted by a message saying '"So and so" has left the meeting'. This ensures that everyone knows who they are speaking to, and prevents anyone from dialling in and eavesdropping without the others' knowledge.

The chair of the conference (who may or may not be the chair of the group) has a separate code. Until this code is entered, other members who have dialled in will hear holding music and a message. Once the chair has joined, all members are announced, and are able to hear each other.

Managing the teleconference

The only way to prevent an unmoderated teleconference descending into chaos is to have a strong chair and rigid rules. The rules include:

- all participants must be in quiet locations (no mobiles on trains or out of doors callers, as background noises are magnified on the call)
- participants must not be doing two things at once (reading emails, making tea – because of background noise and the need to concentrate)
- contributions should be clearly spoken, brief and to the point
- if any members don't know each other, and so wouldn't recognise voices, participants should say who they are whenever they make a comment

The chairperson needs to:

- check that everyone has, and is looking at, the right papers
- ensure that people speak in turn and don't interrupt each other
- specifically invite contributions from people who don't volunteer comments
- prompt people to look at the appropriate page, paragraph or bullet point on papers, in the absence of visual cues
- say clearly when the meeting is over so that people know when to end their calls.

Videoconferencing

Videoconferencing ought to be easier than teleconferencing, because you can at least see the people you are 'meeting', and pick up visual cues. But somehow this doesn't often prove to be the case. In a videoconference, two or sometimes three locations are linked by cameras and an open telephone line so that each group of people sitting at their table can see the other(s) on a large screen, and hear what they say. The quality of systems varies, with some suffering from a slight time delay in transmitting sound, microphones that pick up as much background noise as voices, and a tendency to show jerkily moving pictures of the far site. These add to the difficulties of having meaningful conversations and doing effective business. Better systems have speakers that will only allow one voice to be transmitted at a time, so preventing people speaking over each other, and other tricks such as linked overhead projectors, so that an acetate written and produced at one end can be viewed instantly at the other. However, in my experience of videoconferencing, in a variety of different organisations, the effort required to manage coherent conversation with the far end is so challenging that the simultaneous use of visual aids never crossed our minds!

Good videoconferences need to be effective at getting the business of the groups done, and as brief as possible, both because they are relatively expensive and because they are very demanding on participants.

Key tips to make a videoconference successful

- *Check that you, and everyone at your end of the conference, can be seen by people at the other end*: there is usually an easy way to do this automatically, such as lifting the remote control handset to see an inset picture of 'your end' from 'their end' on the video screen. The camera pointing at you can be made to zoom in or out, or pan round, using the handset so that everyone is included in the picture – but unless you have been shown how to do this, it is best not to experiment! Move the chairs rather than the camera.
- *Keep papers and files away from the desk-top microphones*: they make a great deal of noise at the other end if they are rustled.
- *Speak up, speak clearly and a little slower than usual*: between background noise, transmission quality and time delays, the people at the far end need all the help they can get to make out what you are saying.
- *Look at the screen at all times when speaking*: if you look at people in your own room, you are effectively cutting off the people at the other end, as well as making it more difficult for them to hear you.
- *Don't have sotto voce conversations with people next to you, or pass them notes*: not only will the noise be picked up by the microphones, but remember the people at the other end have a close-up view of what you are doing, and will wonder what you are up to.
- *Try to ignore interruptions in your room*: there is nothing more irritating to the other end than to suddenly see all heads swivel and business cease as something happens that they can't see. The exception to this of course is the fire alarm – and I have known several videoconferences come to a premature end when one set of people had to troop out of the building in mid-flow!
- *Make your contributions short and to the point, and only in response to an invitation from the chair*: it is very difficult to control proceedings if people at both ends

try to speak and interrupt each other, particularly when there is a time delay on transmission.

Online meetings

There are programmes that can enable people sitting at their own computers to link in to a virtual meeting with numerous others. Each person can hear the others (or, without audio, write messages in real time), as well as sharing access to document files and seeing online sketches of diagrams produced during the meeting. Tick box surveys can gather instant views from participants and 'emoticons' can be used to express how people feel about a proposal.

The only way to prepare for one of these meetings is to be formally taught how to use the system by the programme provider, and companies that offer this form of meeting service also run online training seminars. You are unlikely to be invited to participate as an 'outsider', so if your organisation does not have this facility, you needn't worry about this particular advance just yet!

Leaving a group

There is bound to come a time when you feel it is right for you to leave a group or network. This may be because your role, interests or circumstances have changed, or because the group is failing to meet your needs (or failing generally). The worst way to do this is simply to fade away: not attend meetings, and ignore emails. It is much better to exit gracefully with a letter or email to the group chair, secretary or organiser, explaining that you will not be part of the group any more and, if you give a reason, doing so neutrally and courteously. It takes only a little more time and effort, but will leave a much better impression with an important group of people. Remember, you may meet them again one day, and you want them to remember you with respect.

One reason to consider leaving a group is when you find that you are seriously concerned about ideas or actions they are taking forward. There is of course much you can do inside the group to try to influence them away from something you think may be wrong, unethical or unprofessional (not just something you disagree with). But if they are set on doing something that you cannot condone or be associated with, bear in mind that it may not work to remain in the group while disowning a particular part of its work. Unless there is a very clear procedure for recording your dissenting view, the distinction may not be visible to others, and you will be considered to have collaborated in the action by your membership of the group. In this case, you should consider leaving instead. There is no need to throw a tantrum – you can still exit gracefully with an objective and considered explanation. But the letter you write becomes even more important if you wish to be clear that you were not part of the group when it proceeded with the action you object to.

CHECKLIST FOR ACTION

Have you:

- decided how you are going to get the best from each of the groups you currently belong to – which may mean leaving some, or changing the way you work with others?
- if you don't belong to any groups, looked around for an appropriate forum to join?

CHAPTER 21

Making presentations

The biggest visual aid is yourself! (SUE BORAN)

Making a presentation these days is like driving a car: almost everyone finds they have to do it, no matter how much they would prefer not to. They are often left to develop their own skills after minimal training, and frequently acquire bad habits that vary from mildly irritating to outrageous. For some, being asked to make a presentation to a room full of people is like having to drive round the M25 when you normally only drift to the shops in third gear on Sundays if it isn't raining.

The good news is that there are some basic guidelines to effective presentations that can be applied in almost any situation, and which will make you feel much more confident. For those already brimming with confidence, who love to stand up and make a presentation – it is always worth checking that you haven't developed any bad habits. If you distract, irritate or alienate your audience, you will radically diminish the amount of influence you will have over them.

MIRROR MOMENT

Be honest – what kind of a presenter are you? Are you nervous and glad when it's over? Or really confident and a bit complacent, leaving preparation to the last minute, and apologising for your slides or your delivery because you use the same presentation for different audiences? In either case, look objectively at the following guidelines, and be prepared to change your style and make a fresh start.

Opportunities to make a presentation

Making a presentation is just about unavoidable these days. It is common to have to do so as part of a job interview, or when applying for an award. People providing updates on a project or piece of work at a meeting are often expected to do so by giving a presentation rather than simply speaking. And as you become an expert in your clinical area, complete a project, finish some research or get invited to policy-making forums, you are bound to be asked to make a presentation about your subject at some point.

This chapter aims to help you ensure that you give confident, effective presentations, which will enhance your reputation and credibility, without too much stress on your part. Whatever kind of presentation you are giving, in whatever setting, the key is to pay equal attention to three key stages:

- preparation
- planning
- delivery.

Preparation

> *Preparation and contingency planning: have all the modes of presentation with you, trust nobody to provide you with equipment unless you have it in writing.* (Maureen Williams)

The first step in preparing for the presentation is to find out exactly what is required from you. Sounds simple, but it can require some persistence to elicit from the organisers of the meeting, event or conference exactly what they have in mind. It is essential that you know:

- *how long you have for the presentation*: if the answer is vague ('oh, about 15–20 minutes, I should think . . . if that's okay . . .?'), check again nearer the time. The slot may well have changed as other speakers or items on the agenda come and go. It is better to double-check than be caught out with too much or too little material. Check also whether that is all the time available to you (so you might want to leave 5 minutes of it for questions), or if there will be additional time for questions afterwards
- *what the purpose of your presentation is*: are you giving an update, presenting new information, defending an unpopular decision, consulting people? This will influence not only what you say, but how you say it. Treat the information you are given by the organisers with caution: they may say 'it's just to update people on the progress of the project' while knowing perfectly well that the audience is coming along to vent their fury at the changes the project has caused to their working patterns. A presentation at an interview is likely to be at least as much an opportunity for the panel to judge your personal impact, resilience under pressure and presentation skills as it is to hear what you have to say on the topic given. Make your own judgement, with information from different sources if necessary
- *what is the title they have given to your presentation*: it is surprising how often speakers give a talk that doesn't seem to match the title in the programme or on the agenda. If you don't want to give the talk they are asking for, negotiate a change of title or adapt your plans. It is unfair to the audience to wrong-foot

them by talking about something else, and they will blame you rather than the organisers. If events put a different slant on things and you need to change the title, or adapt your talk, close to the date of the event, contact the organisers as soon as possible. It is usually possible to change the paperwork, and better to have this minor inconvenience beforehand than major embarrassment on the day

- *the size and make-up of the audience*: these factors are key to the planning of your presentation, and you should get as much detail as you can. You will want to say different things to a multidisciplinary audience compared to your own professional group; and say them in a different way to an audience of 15 than an audience of 50. Omitting this preparation has caused me major embarrassment in the past: speaking to an audience that included the media when I wasn't expecting them; to an audience of 25 when I had had been told there would be 100+; and to a group that included GPs when I was expecting only practice staff. Again, don't necessarily take the information you are given by the organisers at face value. Check on numbers attending (especially a conference) several times as the date approaches. If it is a meeting, you could check who has sent apologies so that you know who won't be there: just as important if you are bracing yourself to face all the consultants. With regard to the press, it is as well, whatever the organisers tell you, to assume that someone from the media will be in the room at any conference
- *the level of knowledge of the audience*: there is nothing more excruciating than a presenter telling an audience things they already know. It makes the presenter very uncomfortable as the audience grows restless, indignant and bored; and the audience, as ever, tends to blame the presenter even if the fault lies with the organisers who briefed them. You need to know what level of knowledge or experience you should assume before you even start planning your presentation
- *the context for your presentation*: the 'internal context' is important: is this the first presentation of the meeting/event, or will you be facing an audience that has had four other presentations already and is fixated on the forthcoming coffee break? Who are the other speakers, and how does your subject fit in with theirs? You should also keep an eye on the external context: policy announcements, news headlines, relevant professional developments that impact on the area you are about to talk about. It may be unfair, but the audience will expect you to be up to date and able to incorporate these, even if they happened last week and you sent in your presentation, as requested by the organisers, two weeks ago
- *technical limitations*: there is a tendency to assume that the rest of the world is at roughly the same technological level as ourselves. But it is worth checking that the venue for the meeting or event has the kind of equipment you are expecting – and can use. It may only have an overhead projector, not a 'PowerPoint®' projector. There may or may not be microphones. You may be required to take your own laptop for a presentation, or to take your presentation saved on a particular storage device: floppy disk, CD ROM or mass storage device ('memory stick'). Conference organisers, and some meeting organisers, increasingly expect an electronic presentation to be emailed to them in advance, cutting down the

time you have to prepare. In contrast, some interviewers are now asking for presentations delivered with no visual aids at all, in reaction, no doubt, against excessive use of computer presentation packages
- *what other supporting materials you need to supply*: even if your presentation is relatively informal, you may need to provide copies of key points, or a project plan to which you will refer. If you use an electronic presentation, organisers may expect it to be emailed so that they can copy it to delegates. In a meeting, it is useful to have copies to pass round so that people don't struggle to take notes. Whatever you are providing, sending it to the organisers in advance not only means that it can be given to participants efficiently with other papers, it means that you don't have to carry lots of copies to the event.

Planning

The traps

> *Know your audience, and pitch it right. Don't go for a Hollywood extravaganza if it's a local divisional meeting.* (Alison Norman)

Once you know the answers to the questions above, you are in a position to plan a presentation that will be appropriate, targeted, and of the right length and level for your audience and the event. At this point you need to avoid the four worst sins of presenters:
- information overload
- technology overload
- whimsy overload
- ego overload.

> *Keep the slides short and uncluttered, no more than four points a slide. Don't read the slide – talk around the bullet points and be passionate about what you are talking about: your enthusiasm and belief in the topic will come across.* (Judith Whittam)

Too much information simply overwhelms an audience and makes them irritable. Too much on one slide is a common mistake – how many times have you heard a presenter say 'I know this slide is a bit crowded . . .' or 'You may not be able to read this but it doesn't matter . . .' It does matter! Keep as few words on the slide (or acetate) as possible, to act as a prompt for you, and use your own notes if necessary to expand on them. If your presentation is oral, without visual aids, then people have even less chance of keeping up if you give them a large amount of information. If you are only speaking, plan a minimum number of very clear messages, and say them several times if necessary to ensure that they are heard. Accompany your presentation with the offer of a summary paper, or written notes, made at the beginning of your presentation, so that people know they don't have to remember everything or write it all down. This will enable them to relax and focus on what you are saying.

Too much technology is becoming a more common complaint. Many people have never overcome their fascination with the facility of computerised presentation software to add the sound of a speeding bullet or a Venetian blind effect to incoming slides, and to incorporate video clips and music. Presentations that feature numerous graphics and photographs can become bewildering to the audience, who don't know what to expect next and cannot absorb the amount of information on display. It is also difficult, unless you are in your own venue and very familiar with the equipment, to move between different technologies in the same presentation. Keeping the presentation as simple as possible will make the experience easier and less stressful for you, as well as for the audience.

Whimsy overload is to be avoided at all costs. Pictures of your children or pets, verses of poetry and uplifting quotations may have a place occasionally. But generally, playing it straight is more professional and more effective. This applies especially in a situation where the judgement people make about you during your presentation is key to the outcome: for instance, in interviews for jobs or awards. If the audience thinks you are a bit daffy at a conference, it may not affect your future in any way. If the interviewers' toes are curling, you may be talking yourself out of a job you really wanted.

Too much ego often leads directly into the three traps above. If you give people information just to show how much you know, they will spot it. If you use complicated technological effects to demonstrate your grasp of gadgetry, they will either resent it because they can't do it, or deride you because they can do more. And if you make them cringe because you're up there speaking and you have the opportunity to inflict your taste on them, they will not remember another word you say.

Planning to succeed

> *Keep the presentation simple and straightforward – any idiot can bamboozle an audience with jargon and ill-thought out ideas; it takes a clever person to get over complex issues simply.* (Rosalynde Lowe)

So, avoiding all the traps above, how should you decide the nature and content of your presentation? The key is to ask yourself, given what you have found out about the audience, and the occasion:

- what will *most impress* this audience?
- what would be the *best, most simple approach* for this audience?

It may be that what will most impress are some hard facts and figures; or alternatively, demonstrating that you understand their feelings. You may make the best impression by giving them a grand vision of the future; or by putting future plans in practical terms that relate to their workplace. Whatever it is, this should be the focus for your presentation. It is said that audiences retain a maximum of three things they heard during a short presentation: if you build your presentation round the thing that will most impress them, you have some hope that it is that they will remember.

> *Don't be afraid to take risks and use less PowerPoint® and more personal experiences.* (HELEN MOULD)

The simplest approach that will convey this information should be the one you choose. This is not necessarily the most technically simple: if what will most impress them is some killer figures, you may need to use an electronic presentation with a couple of graphs (not too many!) to convey the figures. The simple option of speaking without audiovisual aids might not be the best in this case, as it is difficult for people to compare a lot of figures without something to look at. On the other hand, if you want to convey a vision or win over an audience, speaking directly to the audience, without aids to distract them or you, is often much more effective. Think laterally about your choices: if your subject is how much impact your project has had on patients, you might want to include the voice of a patient in your presentation. This could be:

- with the patient speaking 'live' at the presentation: the most powerful presentation I ever heard on diabetes was from a business man with the condition, who spoke with great emotion of his frustration and anger that he couldn't always keep his blood sugar under control, even with all the gadgets at his disposal
- with a video clip of a patient speaking
- with direct quotes from the patient included on slides, and read by you
- with a patient story told by you. It is noticeable at conferences how much stiller and quieter the audience is when you start to 'tell a story'. Turning away from the laptop, projector or your notes, and speaking directly with a real-life example can be absolutely compelling, and particularly effective in the middle of a more technical presentation.

> *Tune your presentation to the right level – never try to be clever or speak down to audiences.* (KAY EAST)

Having chosen the most simple format for the presentation, confine yourself to including only the most pertinent, effective and impressive material. This is really difficult for some of us, who want to give people everything we have on the subject! But less is almost always more, and definitely so on a projected slide. Have the other information in front of you in notes, so that you can give them more than they can see via the projector or your meeting paper, and to help you answer questions.

Finally in planning your presentation:

- *check your facts* – or someone is bound to catch you out
- *rehearse it and time it*, so that you don't either end up desperately asking the audience to talk among themselves because you have finished in half the time allocated, or get cut off by the chair when you are 15 minutes over time and people are beginning to rebel openly – I have seen both happen!
- *allow time to review and revise your presentation before you finalise it*: so start in good time. Preparing something the day before will not make a good presentation. And if you have had to send it in to the meeting or conference organisers for copying

and distribution, or inclusion in delegate packs, don't then change it! Remember, including minimal trigger information on the slides or notes makes it easier for you to adapt what you say to be up-to-the-minute, without confusing and annoying the audience trying to follow the original version.

Delivering your presentation

Practise, prastise, prastise – be able to deliver without reading from notes.
(SUZANNE HILTON)

The equipment

You will do yourself an enormous favour if you spend a few minutes learning how to operate the various kinds of equipment used in presentations, and what to do when it goes wrong. Not only will this make your presentation run smoothly, and minimise the length of any interruptions, but it adds to the impression you want to convey of someone in control. The audience wants to feel in safe, confident hands, and there is something very awkward about a speaker who stands looking helpless and confused because they can't move a slide on or focus a picture, or make the video player work. So when you know what kind of equipment you will use, if you have any doubts, ask someone who is good at this sort of thing to give you a quick tutorial well before your presentation. Often this need not be a person from the IT department, just a colleague who has more experience. Some of the basics you should know are shown in the 'need to know' Box 21.1.

BOX 21.1 Need to know: presentation equipment

- *Overhead projectors*: how to adjust the size and focus of the image; how to change the bulb if necessary; where to switch it on and off.
- *Projectors and laptops*: how to load your disk, CD ROM or 'memory stick' into the computer, depending which you use; how to find your presentation, open it and start the 'show'; how to move forwards and backwards through the slides; what to do if the screen blanks out; ideally, how to connect the cables that link the projector to the laptop.
- *Video players*: where start, stop, fast forward, rewind and volume controls are, both on the machine and the remote control (if there is one).
- *Microphones*: where the on/off switch is; how far away from your mouth you should hold it; what you should do if you get 'screeching' from interference.

On the day of the presentation, try to get time with the equipment before the audience or meeting participants arrive to check that it is now familiar, and your slides, videotape or whatever are ready to go. Some organisers of major professional conferences offer a whole session to their speakers, showing them how to prepare their presentation and operate the equipment, how to use microphones, what to do if they need help, and so on. If offered, these are definitely worth taking up, no matter how much you think you already know. At a minimum you will usually be shown the equipment and how to do the basics by the audiovisual technician supporting the conference: ask them any questions you have, and get them to show you if you are unsure. They are experts, and very used to nervous speakers – and you will never meet them again, so there is no need to be embarrassed. It is an opportunity for a free, private tutorial, and should be grasped willingly!

Microphones will usually only be available for conference presentations, though there are some formal committees that use table-top microphones. Using microphones can be daunting, and speakers sometimes try to decline them, claiming that they have a loud voice, or will speak up. Don't do this. If microphones are there, it is because the organisers know that the acoustics of the room require it, and you will only irritate both the organisers and the audience if you try to deliver your presentation without it. Even a smallish room may require the use of a microphone when it is full of people. Useful tips are:

- *table microphones*: if these are shared, turn the microphone towards you and speak to it from a distance of around 15 cm. You can usually judge from what you hear of your own voice whether this distance is working, and adjust accordingly. In any case, watch the reaction of the chair and/or members of the audience to see if they indicate a problem. Don't turn your head away while you are speaking, to look round the audience, or your voice will fade in and out. Try not to gesticulate too much, as the noise of touching or brushing the microphone will be horribly amplified for the audience
- *lectern microphones*: if there is only one, and it is to one side of the lectern, you need to be careful not to turn away to look at the audience on the opposite side while speaking, as your voice will fade out. Look at them during a pause, but speak to the microphone. Often there are microphones on each side, and if you stand centrally in front of the lectern you are freer to look around – but not to wave your hands! You don't need to worry about distance from the microphone, as this is dictated by the size of the lectern. If you are particularly tall or small, you may need to move the microphone slightly to pick up your voice, if this isn't done for you
- *lapel microphones*: these are the 'mobile microphones' that clip on to a lapel or tie, and have a wire running to a small black box. Ideally this can be slipped into a jacket pocket, so it is worth remembering to wear such an item. If not, you can slip it inside a waistband, or even hold it in one hand – but this is awkward and best avoided. For best effect, clip the microphone as centrally as possible (on a tie, or shirt/blouse front) – if it is on one lapel, you have the problem of fading out when you look away from the centre line. Make sure it is not fixed so that it can touch a brooch or badge if you raise your arm, as every contact will be amplified. Avoid touching the microphone, a badge or other jewellery such as a necklace while speaking (common nervous habits) for the same reason. Once the microphone is attached, and the black box stowed somewhere, you need to turn the microphone on to speak – there is usually a sliding on/off switch on the top of the transmitter. It is also important to turn it off as soon as you have finished speaking, to avoid the audience hearing comments between you and the next

speaker, chair or organiser, and so that you don't deafen them with the scratching and scrunching as you unclip the microphone and hand it over

- *roving microphones*: these are possibly the most abused of microphones. They are often used for question and answer sessions with an audience, or for *ad hoc* comments – and people generally react as if they have been handed a live rattlesnake. Again, people often try to refuse them, or start to speak without them, but in any crowded meeting or conference room, they are essential. The essential tips are: wait for the microphone; if necessary, turn it on using the sliding on/off switch (either on the bottom of the microphone or the front where your thumb is); hold it very close to your mouth – almost touching your lips – and keep it there; speak normally; turn it off or hand it back when you have finished speaking – don't put it on the table or in your lap while it is still on, while you listen to the response.

Overhead projectors may be dusty items in the basement in some places, but they are still offered for speakers to use in others. With computerised presentations much more common, it worth reminding yourself of some key tips for using overhead projectors effectively, in case you need to use one (*see* Box 21.2).

BOX 21.2 Tips for overhead projector presentations

- *Make sure your acetates are clean*: bits of fluff, fingerprints and dusty smears will be projected onto the screen along with the writing.
- Check before you start that you have somewhere to put down the acetates you are about to use, and those you have finished with, in two separate piles, to avoid messy fumbling.
- If it is the first time you are using them, separate the acetate from the protective paper gummed to it before you do your presentation; keep the paper between the acetates to stop them sticking to each other, but spare the audience the ripping sound between every slide.
- *Practise placing the first acetate on the projector before you start*, if possible, to check the best position to put it to get the whole thing on the screen: then you will be more confident at placing the others without a lot of adjustment.
- *Don't talk while you are trying to position the acetate*: get it in the right place, then look up and talk.
- *Don't talk over your shoulder to the screen*: take one quick look to check the slide is correctly positioned, then face the audience, reading from the acetate if necessary, not the screen.
- *Don't use handwritten acetates*: they will always look amateurish, and as slides can be prepared on computer and printed out onto acetates, there is no excuse.

One other simple but essential piece of equipment to remember is a watch – or even a clock. You need a way to keep an eye on the time while you are speaking: a watch will do for a meeting but may be difficult to focus on when presenting in a larger arena, and you can't be sure there will be a wall clock. Some people take a small alarm clock to sit on the lectern or speaker's table. If you are worried about trying to monitor yourself while you are speaking, you can always ask the chair of the meeting or conference to give you a five minute warning before your time is up. As it is entirely in their interests that the event runs to time, they will be only too pleased to do so.

You

> *Power dress, or feel good about how you look – 'confidence dress'.* (Judith Ellis)

Mastering the technology will make you look and feel more confident: how you proceed to deliver your presentation needs to match this image. Experienced presenters are often surprisingly nervous before delivering a presentation, even in informal settings with fewer people. Few people are so self-confident that they don't worry that people will judge them harshly on their performance. So practising some simple habits can help:

- take some deep breaths just before you are introduced and consciously relax your muscles

> *Everyone in the world gets nervous, it's expected and it'll pass.* (Sandra Mellors)

- smile brilliantly before you start: at the chair, the audience or the previous speaker – it doesn't matter who, but it will relax your throat and face and make it easier to speak. Smiling at the audience is always a good idea!
- look round the whole audience or meeting table at the beginning, while you say 'thank you for inviting me' or 'I'm delighted to be here' or whatever is appropriate – you will feel more confident for having seen them, rather than pretending they are not there
- some people start with a joke or light-hearted comment, or a cartoon on their first slide, as a smile or laugh from the audience puts both parties at ease – but this can feel forced, and there is nothing worse than a stony-faced response if it doesn't work! Test a few ways of getting started to find what works best for you

> *never say how nervous you are, how you don't really know much about the topic, how you haven't had enough time to prepare, how the after-lunch slot is the graveyard slot and everyone is sure to fall asleep . . .* (Rosalynde Lowe)

- if you are unsure that the minimalist 'prompt' words or diagrams on the slides will remind you of what you need to say, you can have some further prompts in front of you, on a printed-out version of the slides or a set of index cards. Staple or otherwise fix them together so that they can't slip off the lectern or table and get muddled up. These sorts of prompts work better at a meeting table, when glancing down is easy and looks more natural, than at a lectern, when it is hard to change your focus constantly between the far reaches of the audience and your handwriting on your notes. If possible, rehearse your presentation sufficiently, and choose your prompt words or diagrams carefully, so that you can speak without any further notes

- face forward – to the audience – at all times: resist the temptation to speak over your shoulder to the projection screen, or down to your paper. If you want to check something, pause while you look at it, then look up and deliver it. As we all tend to speak much more quickly when we are nervous or self-conscious, this has the useful effect of slowing down your delivery, and makes what you say when you look up have all the more impact

> *Make eye contact with your audience straight away, whatever its size – even if you can't see them through the lights you need to look as if you can. Look as if you want to be there with them even if you don't!* (Sue Norman)

- have a closing sentence prepared. Even if you are good at speaking off the cuff to your slides or notes, the confident effect can be spoilt if you come to a sudden halt, or say lamely 'That's it really . . . er . . .'. Plan a final few sentences that summarise what you have said, say 'thank you' firmly and make eye contact with the chair. He or she will then take over and lead the applause, invite questions, or move on to the next item, as appropriate.

If you approach your presentation well prepared, and put into practice the tips above, you will not only give effective presentations, but rapidly become known as a 'good speaker' and be invited to speak more regularly. Why? Because so many people ignore or break these simple guidelines, and in doing so create problems for people around them: their audience, the chair, and the event organisers.

I chaired a conference recently which had a very good programme, with a series of very interesting presentations from a wide range of speakers of all levels of experience. It was basically a well-designed, well-organised event. But in the course of one session we had a speaker who arrived in the hall two minutes before she was due to speak, with her presentation on a memory stick to be loaded; another who finished nearly 10 minutes before her allotted time; and several who arrived in the hall but failed to let the chair or organisers know they were there. We had speakers looking over their shoulders at the screen, moving away from the microphone, not bringing (or sending in advance) copies of their presentation, and filling their allotted time then inviting audience questions. There was one who insisted on getting the audience to stand up and do an exercise first, and one who had far too many slides, filled with far too much information, and 'fast-forwarded' through them because he was 'aware of the time'. This is not unusual – and why you should never assume the chair's job is an easy one!

Remember, a good speaker is not necessarily a brilliant orator, inspirational guru or major wit. It is one who:

- prepares well
- arrives in good time
- delivers useful material with conviction
- finishes on time
- handles the ending well (and the question and answer session – *see* below).

A good speaker is also someone who doesn't:

- repeat their name and title when they have just been introduced
- read out verbatim what is written on each slide
- apologise for the slides/information/readability
- wander about or fidget
- run away afterwards so that people can't speak to them.

When things go wrong . . .

The nightmares that people have before they do a presentation usually feature all the things that could go wrong: the slides won't move on, you're going on too long, you run out of things to say too soon, the audience starts heckling, you choke on a fly, you look down and realise you're naked . . . Apart from the last one, these things will undoubtedly happen to you at some time if you speak regularly, so it's a good idea to have some techniques ready to handle them.

If the slides won't move on (or back) when you want them to – try to pre-empt this by having your presentation loaded onto the computer before the meeting or event starts, and asking the technician (at a conference) or meeting organiser to show you how to move them on and back. At the same time you can confirm with them what you should do if there is a problem when you are presenting: they may show you a trick to do yourself, or tell you to leave it to them to sort from the control box. If it does happen, don't get embarrassed and comment on it: it draws attention, and distracts you from the thread of your talk. If following the instructions you were given doesn't work, make eye contact with the technician, organiser or chair, and ask for someone to help. If they appear straightaway you can wait for the next slide. If not, pick up your notes and talk directly to the audience. The worst thing to do is let a long pause develop, while you vacillate about whether to go on and the audience becomes restless. Appearing in control (even if you don't feel it) reassures the audience and keeps their attention.

If you are over-running your time, or you realise that you are likely to over-run – some people flick rapidly through their slides, or turn over several pages of notes, for the reassurance of reaching the end and 'completing' the presentation. I think this gives a poor impression, as it demonstrates clearly to the audience that you have not timed your presentation well. An alternative approach is to leave the slide you have reached up, or put down your notes, and summarise, strongly and confidently, your main message. Then smile, say thank you and handover to the chair. This gives a strong finish, and leaves a good impression of you as a speaker – some people will never notice that they didn't get all of your slides! If you think it will be obvious, because you have provided a handout of your notes or slides, you can still pretend that all is well by acknowledging these: 'There are other examples in my paper, that you might want to refer to later' you can say magnanimously. Or 'I have listed the various stages of the project on later slides, and you have these in your handout – but I want to leave you with a quote from one of our service users . . .'

If you are running out of material but still have significant time in hand, you have several options. If the programme or meeting is over-running, you could finish early, without remarking on it, and help the programme to catch up. However, it is generally not helpful to the chair and organisers to simply finish early if the programme is running to time – the next speaker may not be ready, refreshments or lunch may not be in place, and it makes their programme look 'thin' – so don't assume you are doing them a favour. If you have time to fill before the next speaker's slot, you could finish and say 'I wanted to leave time for questions, so I'll stop there . . .' Or you could fill the time by summarising what you have said into a strong finish; or by diverting from your presentation to tell a relevant patient's story, or to describe an element of your subject in more detail. The change of pace can actually improve the presentation, and earn you a good evaluation from grateful listeners.

If the audience starts misbehaving – this is a very scary moment! Check if it is due to something you can control: is your microphone working, can they hear you, can they see the slides? Sometimes just pausing to ask these things is enough to shame chattering or restless people into settling down to listen. Make lots of eye contact, across the whole room, and smile to keep yourself relaxed. If problems continue, you could pause and look across – but I feel it is generally not a good idea to say anything about the interruption. This makes the rest of the audience squirm, breaks your thread and makes the people you embarrass in this way *really* hostile. If behaviour is bad enough to need to be addressed explicitly – barracking, taking mobile phone calls – then the chair of the event should take control and stop it. You do the quiet dignity while they do the head teacher!

If you choke on a fly – or start spluttering for any other reason – don't press on regardless. It's difficult for you, deafens the audience if you are using a microphone, and will only get worse with the embarrassment. If no-one offers you a glass of water, ask for one.

If you look down and find you are naked – you're probably asleep, so don't worry about it.

Handling a question and answer session

Read the audience and flex to their feedback. (Fran Woodard)

This can be more nerve-wracking than making the presentation – and arguably if it isn't, it should be. This is dangerous territory: having had a chance to prepare and rehearse the presentation, you are suddenly required to think on your feet at the point when you are just relaxing because the formal part is over. This is often the moment when something embarrassing, confidential or just plain silly pops out of your mouth before you can stop it. Beware of the three Bs: burbling, blundering and blagging.

- *Burbling* is the tendency to talk too much in response to a question because you can't think of a sensible answer. Audiences and chairs hate it, and it should be avoided at all costs.
- *Blundering* is letting out a piece of information or opinion you didn't mean to share, usually because you are provoked by an aggressive question, or seduced by a friendly one. Journalists love this, which is why it is another major trap to avoid.
- *Blagging* is making up figures, findings or, worse, whole policies, on the hoof because you don't know the right answer and you don't want to admit it. There are alternatives, and you should always use them.

To avoid these traps, try the following:

- *note down the questioner's name and where they are from when they give it*: this allows you to think whether you know anything in their locality (project, good practice, good contact) that you can refer to in your answer
- *note down the gist of the question*: this can be difficult because questions are sometimes very long and rambling, and may include more than one issue or request. If you are not sure what they really want to know, jot down one element of the question, and repeat it back to them before answering it: 'you mentioned our pay scales for the new roles; I'll tell you how we approached this . . .'
- *acknowledge questions that are not really questions*, rather than try to answer them – some people in meetings or at conferences will use the invitation to ask a question as a chance to rant a bit and let off steam about the subject. If there is no question to answer, don't try. Acknowledge politely ('That's an interesting viewpoint', 'Thank you, I will let the steering group know how you feel') and wait for the next question
- *keep your answers short and concise*: don't repeat elements of your presentation. Less is more in this situation, as there are probably other people who would like a chance to ask a question too. Better to answer several different questions than just one
- *be polite and positive, whatever the provocation*. If the questioner is rude, insulting, patronising or ranting – or if the question is just plain stupid – it is tempting to use your time with the mirophone, your position on the stage, and your hard-won knowledge and expertise, to slap them down. It is easy to make the questioner look silly, to turn the audience against them or to demonstrate your superior status. But it leaves a bad impression of you with the rest of the audience – which, remember, may well include people from the press and future contacts you would like to make, as well as the other speakers and the chair. So grit your teeth, smile, and handle the question graciously. Useful phrases are:
  - I realise you feel strongly about this – perhaps we could talk about it after the session?
  - I have noted what you say

   - I don't think I'm going to convince you . . .
   - perhaps we should agree to differ and move on
- If things get really difficult, the chair should intervene. If this doesn't happen, you can always say firmly 'Next question?' and fix your gaze firmly on the chair, or another part of the audience. Don't pursue an argument to try to reach agreement: remember there are other people who want their chance to ask questions
- if you are on a panel, it is even more important not to take up too much time. Keep answers even briefer, and if you don't have a contribution to make in response to a question, don't speak for the sake of it. Simply say you have nothing to add, with a complimentary smile to the other panel members to acknowledge how clever they have been
- if you are really concerned about getting a bad reaction to your presentation – and you can usually anticipate this, if you have done your preparation – then it is worth trying to anticipate the questions or challenges that will follow, and preparing some answers and points to make in advance.

BOX 21.3 Abstracts for conferences

All the guidance that you need is supplied by the conference organisers in the 'call for papers' or 'call for abstracts' – but often there are papers that miss out because people overlook or ignore the guidelines. So:

- check you are targeting the right conference by looking at the aims set out, and the wording of the invitation to submit papers/abstracts
- follow the instructions to the letter, especially regarding word length, information to be included and deadline for submissions
- take time to rewrite and refine so that it is a small but perfectly formed piece of work in its own right – this indicates to the organisers that you will give equal care and consideration to a full presentation, so treat it as a mini-paper
- keep the conference audience in mind as you word your abstract: organisers are used to submissions about a piece of research or a project that is desperately looking for a platform. You need to convince them that their particular audience will want to hear about *this* piece of work by pointing out the relevance it has for them
- use all the best impact information you have in the abstract: rather than blandly asserting that the experience of your project will enthuse the audience, give some of the measurable outcomes that will 'wow' them. It is like a trailer for a film: it often contains all the best bits, but people still want to see the film because they loved the trailer and they hope that there is more of the same in the full-length version!

PORTFOLIO POINTER

It is a good idea to start a list in your portfolio of your presentations to conferences, groups and other significant audiences. List the nature of the presentation (platform, workshop), the title, audience size and make-up and so on. As you do more of them, it is easy to forget where you have been and what you have done, but you might want to summarise, or give specific instances, on a job application, or to demonstrate your experience when putting in an abstract for another conference (*see* Box 21.3 for more on abstracts). One way to do this is to keep a copy of the conference programme which features your name and presentation details in your portfolio. This has the advantage of putting your presentation into context, as well as proving that you are not making it all up in a Walter Mitty-like fantasy! You might also want to keep a copy of some of your presentations, and check back from time to time to ensure that your skill and style has developed, and you are not simply reproducing the same look and content year after year.

CHECKLIST FOR ACTION

Have you:

- reviewed your presentation technique to check for bad habits?
- put in an abstract to a relevant conference?

CHAPTER 22

Influence at conferences

Consider your persona, i.e. body language, dress sense, ability to enunciate words and general bearing. (ALEXANDRA LEJEUNE)

Conferences are the most expensive and commonly wasted influencing opportunities in the professional calendar. Few care workers would consider throwing away several hundred pounds' worth of clinical equipment or office supplies, and they would expect to be disciplined if they did. But some seem content to waste the same sort of sum when it has been spent on a place at a conference. They attend only the sessions on their favourite or familiar topics; they speak only to the colleagues they came with, and spend the lunch break hunched over their mobile phone; they tour the exhibition only to pick up some freebies, if at all; then leave early to go shopping or catch the early train home. Few people will do all of these things at one conference, but many people are guilty of one or two, and can be breathtakingly blatant about it.

Apart from squandering the money spent on their place at the conference, these people are also wasting a prime opportunity to increase their awareness and exercise their influence. A day spent constructively at a conference can lead to new contacts, involvement in new pieces of work, opportunities to write, speak or make presentations, or simply registering on the radar of someone who, in future, will remember you and want your contribution to a piece of work.

I remember very clearly the first national conference that I went to. It was the Association of Primary Care Facilitators annual conference and AGM, in Harrogate. There were only about 30 people there, and a tiny exhibition. But, almost by accident rather than design, I came away with a place on the executive of the Association, a commission for an article for the *Health Visitor* journal, an invitation to contact the director of the then Health Visitors' Association, and a clutch of contact numbers for people doing the same, rather isolated, job as me in different parts of the country. I remember feeling rather dazed by it all: I had always assumed that it would be much harder to get such opportunities. That was the start of my 'external' activities, and many of my current network contacts, and significant parts of my CV, can be traced back to that event.

MIRROR MOMENT

Think about your own approach to a day at a conference. If you tend to keep to yourself and leave as soon as possible, ask yourself what would make it easier for you to do differently next time. Could you make arrangements so that you can take a later train home or arrive earlier? If you wore more comfortable shoes, and didn't carry a heavy case, would you spend more time walking round the exhibition? Could you get your work duties fully covered, so that you don't have to switch on your phone at lunch time? Sometimes the problem is less practical than personal. If you find it hard to speak to people you don't know, or hate going to an event where you don't know anyone, work on this before you go to your next conference. Or decide that, as no-one there will know you, you can leave behind the more reserved version of you, and be someone different for the day!

Choosing the right conference

Choice may seem like a luxury you will never be afforded. But any organisation that is prepared to fund employees' attendance at a conference will want them to get maximum value from it, so you should be able to say why one event will offer you more than another. You might end up being 'sent' to a particular event because 'someone from here has to go', in which case it is important to make the best of it – but where any kind of professional development planning or appraisal goes on, you should expect at least a dialogue about where you go. There are people who pay for their own attendance at conferences, and some even take annual leave to attend. In this case it is even more important that you go to the event that will give you the most for your money.

So how do you choose? Two rules immediately spring to mind:

- always look carefully at the programme before deciding to book a place
- don't go to any conference out of habit, if the programme doesn't look good.

It is easy to feel that, if you are a practice nurse, the best conference for you will be the national practice nurse conference, and similarly for every other group of workers in health and social care. While your 'home' conference may be very good for meeting lots of people doing the same job, it can tend to keep your focus narrow and parochial. Instead, why not aim for a conference that focuses on the service you work in (speech and language therapy, child protection, residential care, or primary care generally), and features speakers from different professions or disciplines who will give a broader view and different opinions. Alternatively, choose an event that meets a particular training need you have identified (new developments in day surgery, the latest on home births, environmental impacts on health), so that you can expect to come away with some clearly identifiable benefit.

Assessing the programme

When checking the programme in order to choose a conference, there are some key things you can look for to assess how much you will get from it:

- *the objectives*: most conference programmes will say what the aims and objectives of the event are. Check they match yours
- *the sessions*: if you want to know about the next steps in non-medical prescribing, but the presentations at the prescribing conference are about new drugs for specific conditions, you will be disappointed. Don't be fooled by a generic title of a conference into booking a place without critically analysing the content of the sessions on offer
- *the speakers*: big names in the field can be good, but maybe you've heard them, or their views, before. Don't be put off by speakers you haven't heard of, with local rather than national jobs: they often present the most interesting sessions based on real experience, and make the most useful new contacts. The best conferences combine both kinds of speaker and both strategic and operational perspectives. Remember you may have a valuable opportunity to speak to them after their presentation
- *the choices*: many conferences have a choice of concurrent sessions, workshops or fringe meetings that allow you to tailor what you hear more closely to your needs – all more value for money!
- *the format*: this needs to match your needs. If you want to network, meet people, and share your ideas, then a conference that is all speeches in the main hall, with no question and answer or panel discussion, will not help you as much as one with workshops, panels or debates. On the other hand, if you want to make a 'big statement' about something, you want an opportunity with the whole audience present. More interactive formats – 'market place' or 'world café' sessions (lots of smaller groups that you can move between, listening and contributing at will) – are good for picking up lots of ideas and contacts
- *added extras*: an exhibition, resources display, 'networking session', internet café, reception, dinner or other additional event can add many more opportunities.

PERSONAL DEVELOPMENT EXERCISE

Practise looking critically at a range of conference programmes, advertised in the journals you read or on flyers or websites. Appraise the speakers, sessions, options, exhibitors etc, for their relevance and interest to you: would they meet any of your learning or development needs? Even if you have no chance of attending, it is a good exercise in developing an analytical approach.

Affording the conference

Many good conferences are expensive, and will take a big chunk out of any training budget. If finding the money to fund conference attendance is a problem, consider:

- putting in an abstract to present a paper, poster or workshop at a conference you know you will want to attend (*see* Box 21.3, p. 165 on preparing an abstract, and Box 22.1 on preparing a poster). Usually this means that you don't pay for your place (though some conference organisers will expect you to pay if you are only bringing a poster), and as a speaker, you should also be able to claim your travel expenses
- building your influence as a writer on a particular topic, with articles in relevant journals (*see* Chapter 17) – you are very likely to be invited to speak on 'your' subject sooner or later, or chair a workshop, and repeat offers will follow. You may never pay to attend a conference again!
- get involved with any national or regional groups relevant to your area of work or background (*see* Chapter 20) – and persuade the group to take an exhibition stand at the conference, or run a workshop or fringe meeting. If you are on the executive committee of the group, this may also help your abstract to be accepted
- offer to share a place with a colleague at a 2–3-day conference, so that your employer's money goes further by contributing to two people's professional updating
- look out for free conferences put on by the Department of Health or agencies relevant to your area of work: these happen surprisingly often when there is a policy message to get over, or when implementation of a policy needs a 'kick-start'
- search out bursaries and educational grants for healthcare workers that can be spent on conference attendance: look in the professional journals, on the internet (especially rdinfo.org.uk), and on university noticeboards.

BOX 22.1 Presenting a poster

This is sometimes seen as the poor relation to being asked to speak at a conference, but it offers you many of the same opportunities. You may get a free, or reduced-price, place at the conference. You will have a chance to be at the conference, attend other sessions, promote your work, meet interested people, and raise your profile as someone connected with your specialist subject.

But anyone who has been at a conference will have seen some dreadful posters, and some shamefully wasted opportunities. To make the most of yours:

- take note of the information given by the organisers about the space available for your poster, whether it has to have a specific orientation (landscape or portrait), and how it will be fixed – a poster that is too big, too small or curling at the edges with inadequate fixings looks unprofessional and will lose attention immediately
- plan what goes onto your poster carefully – and keep it to the minimum. Too many words, complex diagrams, lists of references etc clutter the appearance, and are unreadable to most passers-by. Resist the temptation to put the whole story of your research or project onto the poster. Stick to key facts, and maybe a photograph, quote or chart, that emphasise impact on patients or services: what has changed because of your work? Don't be afraid to limit it to a few key facts – the rest can be passed on by talking to people or supplying copies of a fuller paper that people can pick up if interested

- get help with the preparation and printing of the poster – medical illustration departments of hospitals are often excellent and helpful; the communications manager is an expert on the subject. Really good, well-chosen content can be let down by a poorly designed and printed poster. Try to avoid just printing off a lot of slides to stick up. The cost of a poster is minimal compared to the cost of attending the conference, so try to get funds from your manager, a trust or educational fund, or a sponsor to produce an impressive product. (Remember the poster can be used at other events, and displayed in the trust, practice or home premises afterwards to impress other staff and visitors)
- when the poster is on display at the conference, try to be on hand during breaks to answer questions and make good contacts. Many people simply leave a pile of explanatory papers and business cards, but these are soon left messy and disorganised and detract from the professional image of the poster. Besides, people tend to drift in exhibitions: if you want to really sell your work, you need to be there to snag their attention and engage them in conversation.

PERSONAL DEVELOPMENT EXERCISE

Make it a project to acquire a place at one more conference or event than you would normally manage over the next 12 months, either by finding funding, getting a paper accepted, offering to chair a session or any other (legal) method.

Preparing to attend

So you have the funding and the time agreed to attend a conference, and you have chosen one that matches your needs and ambitions. Rather than sit back and wait, there are some steps you can take before the event to make sure you get the most out of it.

- *Tailor your programme*: decide in advance which sessions you will attend, where there are choices, so that you can think about what exactly you want to learn or contribute on the day. Don't automatically choose your favourite or 'best' topics: try something different, more challenging or presented from a new perspective. Spot the speakers you want to make contact with, and book into their sessions. If someone else from the same organisation is going to the event, make sure you book into different sessions, so that you can share notes and handouts later and double your benefit.
- *Plan your day*: try to arrange travel so that you get to the venue early and do not have to leave early. Much of the benefit from a conference comes from discussions with other delegates in between sessions, and from talking to speakers after their presentation. Leaving early reduces your chance to do this. Try to make arrangements so that you don't have to phone home or the office in the breaks, so that you can use the time more effectively.

- *Set up some meetings outside of the booked sessions*: with people from your regional group or other network whom you don't see often, or with people from national organisations who you think will be there. Be clear what you want from them – to tell them the latest on a new initiative you are leading, put together a joint letter to a journal, or to ask about the organisation's plans on a specific issue. A national conference brings together so many people in the same place, it is an ideal opportunity to do some extra influencing business without additional travel costs or diary time!
- *Plan the best use of the exhibition*: most well-organised national conferences will let you know which organisations will be exhibiting at the event, either through a copy of the programme, or on the conference website. Decide what information you want, and who you really want to speak to, and target their stands specifically. For example:
  - *government departments*: these will often have a stand at a major national conference. You can pick up copies of policy documents, news releases, publications and guidance, and have a chance to speak to officials on the stand. This is a good chance to tell them about your initiatives, ideas or views. Don't expect them to absorb the information in detail in the middle of a conference, but aim to make a good impression, leave them your contact details, and get their email address so you can follow up
  - *company stands*: equipment, training and service companies, and pharmaceutical manufacturers, may be represented. Target them if you want some patient information materials (and are prepared to take those containing their logo), information on the latest gadgets or medicines, or to ask about funding/support for a local event or project
  - *journals*: major and relevant specialist journals often have stands at conferences. This is an ideal opportunity to approach the editor with a well-thought-through article idea. If the editor isn't there in person – and for the specialist journals, they often are – then leave your contact details, an outline of the idea and a good, professional impression, and they may well ring you back. If not, you can of course ring them, with the introduction: 'I spoke to your representative on the stand . . .'
  - *bookshop*: a conference bookshop will often bring together a lot of publications relevant to the audience, and have booklists available from all the major publishers. Bigger conferences may have separate stands for individual publishers of relevant books – this is a great opportunity to find out who you should contact with an idea for a book, or a contribution to a book
  - *professional organisations*: pick up publications and flyers for events, training and awards, and speak to officers about your work or information/resources you need. Again, aim to leave them with an impression of professionalism and courtesy, so that you can build on the contact and go back to them after the conference to develop the relationship.
- *Prepare for new contacts*: it is always worth taking a notebook for jotting down not only who you spoke to, but what you said you would do for them and by when! If

you don't have a supply of business cards to give to new contacts, print out some slips of paper with your details on and take those along instead.

On the day

Once at the event, all that remains is to put your plan into practice. Attend the sessions on time, take brief notes, gather materials from presentations, and visit the stands you identified in the exhibition first, before looking around the others. Don't waste a moment of this expensive opportunity! While waiting for the conference to start, it is a good idea to scan the delegate list provided, and spot people that you would like to meet from their job title, or organisation, or part of the country that they come from. Then you can look out for them via their delegate badges, ask the organisers to pass on a message, or email them afterwards (finding their address by checking their organisation's website) – depending how much you want to pursue them.

Panel sessions/questions and answers

> *Ask questions in plenaries but only if they are thoughtful and short questions.*
> (Deb Lapthorne)

These sessions provide the most direct opportunity to participate in the business of the conference. Many speakers dread them, and with good cause. It is common to face questions that are really well-rehearsed grievances or long rambling expositions of how things are different in X or Y organisation; it is less common to be criticised, hectored or insulted; and not unknown to be petitioned by an audience member invading the stage or slow-hand-clapped by the assembled mob. So the way to stand out as a delegate when participating at such a session is to be courteous, succinct, objective and technically adept.

> *At conferences, be measured and strategic about what you say. Don't just do it from the top of your head, prepare. If you want the speaker to think kindly of you and your organisation, don't put them on the spot.* (Alison Norman)

I recently contacted, and invited to join a national group, a nurse whom I only met once, when she asked a question at a conference. She expressed herself well, showed an understanding of the wider aspects of the subject, handled the inadequate answer graciously, and gave such a good account of her role, that I knew immediately that she would be both valuable and impressive in the group. Asking questions at a conference is undoubtedly a real opportunity to be 'spotted'!

So, what should you do in practice?

- *Be courteous*: this doesn't mean grovelling to the speaker. Lengthy thanks for the brilliance of the presentation only wastes time when other people want to ask questions too. It means smiling, introducing yourself, and framing your question to avoid criticism, or an aggressive approach. Also remember to be courteous to people who aren't there – such as members of other professions, civil servants, journalists and patients. You don't know who is in the audience, who in the audience is related to one of the above, and who will report what you said with great glee the next day.

- *Be succinct*: the questions asked at these sessions can be very lengthy and convoluted, with all sorts of extraneous information, anecdote and personal opinion, until the panel member loses the thread completely and doesn't know what point he/she is supposed to be addressing when the end finally arrives. It is a good idea to note down your question during the session – firstly as vaguely as it occurs to you, then later refined into a coherent sentence. There is usually time for this either during the presentation itself, or immediately afterwards during the applause, assembling of the panel, and introduction to the session. You will see the relief and appreciation on the faces of the speaker and the chair when you offer a question in this form – and simple, straightforward questions have been known to earn a round of applause from an audience!
- *Be objective*: take time, mentally or on paper, to phrase the question in the most neutral way possible. This removes any sense that you are blaming or criticising the speaker, which is both courteous and protects your position: if you ask a question loaded with sarcasm or scepticism, and the response is reasonable and informative, you will look foolish
  - for example: if the speaker has described an innovation in service that they have implemented, and your initial jotted question was '??cost? GPs pay for it??', a poor way to phrase the question would be: 'You said this service cost an extra £20,000 a year for the new post. There's no way our GPs would fork out like that – and they run all the practice-based commissioning groups round our way.' A more neutral question would be: 'Can you tell us how you got the funding for this service agreed?' or 'Could you say more about your approach to the commissioners for funding?'. Prefacing this by acknowledging a positive aspect – 'It sounds like a really good service' – is even better.
- It is just as important to *finish your question courteously and neutrally*: thank the speaker for their answer, however inadequate; if the microphone or opportunity has gone, at least smile at them. If you have the speaker on the ropes, unable to respond to your telling question effectively, the rest of the audience will be well aware of it. You will only gain in kudos from the speaker, the chair and most people in the room if you let them off gracefully, with thanks and a smile, and let them move on. It is rude, and damaging to the impression you give, to pursue the issue or gloat visibly.
- *Be technically adept*: if there is a microphone in use, wait for it to arrive then use it properly. Some people hold it away from them as if it is a live snake, others like a lollipop they have lost interest in, letting it sink gently into their lap while they are speaking. Hold it close to your mouth and keep your head still while speaking. It will usually be given to you already switched on, so you won't need to fiddle

with it, but you will need to keep it away from jewellery or buttons. If you keep hold of it while listening to the answer, keep it still and don't put it down or in your lap while it is still on. Remember that it will pick up any snorts, sniggers or expletives that slip out while you have it in your hand!

> *Ask questions if you get a chance, but if not and you are very keen to meet the speaker, go up to them after the session and make a brief point or ask a short question. Ask if you may email them, then send a follow-up note afterwards. Don't expect results every time – speakers at conferences are usually very busy people.* (Judy Hargadon)

Speaking at a conference

> *If speaking, try and stay for the day or at least until after the next break, e.g. after coffee or lunch – leaving immediately prevents networking and also suggests that you consider your time and therefore your role more important than others'.* (Judith Ellis)

Chapter 15 of this book showed how relatively easy it is to establish yourself as an expert in your subject. With a few articles published, groups joined or projects completed, you are very likely to find yourself a speaker at a conference rather than a delegate. Whether by invitation of the organisers, or by submitting an abstract, sooner or later you will be giving a presentation, leading a workshop or presenting a poster at a conference. For hints on presenting a poster, *see* Box 22.1, p. 170, and for information on preparing and making a presentation, *see* Chapter 21. To make the most of the opportunity and ensure that you get more invitations in future:

- impress the organisers by responding promptly to their requests for information such as a biography and abstract, and copies of your presentation – and certainly by the deadline they give. Arrive early at the venue, and introduce yourself to the organisers so that they know you are there. If you are delayed, ring ahead to let them know so they can make plans to handle it. It is always better for them to know what is happening, however bad the news, than to be left wondering if you will turn up with five minutes to spare, or are 20 miles away in stationary traffic. Speak about what you were asked to speak about (it's amazing how many people change their presentation from the title in the programme, and don't think to tell the organisers) and finish on time
- impress the chair of the session by being in the hall or room in good time, knowing how to use the equipment, delivering well, using the microphone properly and finishing on time
- introduce yourself to the other speakers – it is likely that, as you are speaking at the same conference, these are people who should be in your network. This is a good chance to meet some very senior people who are giving keynote addresses at the conference. Use your business cards/contact detail slips so that they are less likely to forget you when they have thrown away their conference packs

- stay as long as possible – talk to delegates and other speakers after your session and in the breaks, and offer to answer questions afterwards if there is no question and answer session planned. It may feel exhilarating to be the important speaker who has to rush off to do more important things immediately after their presentation – but being accessible, helpful and responsive is far better for you in the long run
- find out which journalists are there, and speak to them to offer to clarify anything you have said – better to help them get it right than find yourself reading a garbled version later. Remember, it is wise to assume that there are always journalists present – and speak accordingly
- dress slightly more formally than you would as a delegate at the conference – it will make you look authoritative and feel more confident. Jackets are not only good for looking formal, they have lapels and pockets for radio microphones.

Handling question and answer sessions

When it is your turn to be answering questions from an audience, you can hope that they follow the tips given earlier – but never count on it. Chapter 21 contains some detailed advice about handling questions after a presentation, while avoiding the three Bs – burbling, blundering and blagging.

When you are attending other conferences, watch and learn from the good examples (and the poor ones) set by other speakers handling questions and answers. For example, some officials from government departments are cautious to the point of inanity in their desire not to let slip anything they shouldn't. Meanwhile, some practitioners are spontaneous to the point of stupidity in sharing their views with the wider world. There is a middle line somewhere, but it is very blurred, and even experienced speakers get it wrong sometimes.

Since you may be misquoted or misremembered, even if you give the ideal answer, there is no point in being unduly paranoid. But it always pays to think twice before making jokes, witticisms or criticisms when you are up there with a microphone. They may make you feel powerful and important at the time, but these unguarded utterances are most likely to give offence.

Chairing a conference session

When you are known for your profile in a particular area, you may be asked to chair a conference or a session rather than speaking at it. Oddly, while everyone recognises the importance of good conference organisers and speakers, people do not always appreciate the skills of a good chair. They can make the difference between a restive, anxious audience, disappointed organisers and flustered speakers – and an event that runs like clockwork without anyone really knowing why. Chairing an event, or a session at an event, is a real skill, but elements of it can be practised and developed.

The chair of a session should be in control, but relatively unobtrusive. They should hear everything, see everything but say as little as possible to keep things on track. Think of the chair as the orchestral conductor, rather than the star soloist, who is expected to cope with everything from a diva in a tantrum to a broken string on a cello without anyone in the audience noticing. As usual there are three key phases to doing a good job of chairing: before, during and after the session or event.

Before the session begins

- Study the programme carefully, so that you know the expected timings, speakers' names, running order, breaks and so on. At the same time, prepare to be flexible, in case someone is late or doesn't appear. Look at the subjects they will speak about, and think whether you could say something to tide over a gap, or if the programme is suitable for you to set up a debate or audience discussion if necessary.
- Check that all your speakers are there in the room before you are due to open proceedings, preferably lined up in the front row so you can keep an eye on them! Introduce yourself to them before the start, check that you know how to pronounce their names, and how they wish to be introduced. Some 'professors' and 'dames' are mortified if you use their full title – some are mortified if you don't! Find out how they want to be prompted about time – do they want a five-minute warning, or a two-minute warning? If they say they don't need a warning because they are so good at timing themselves – agree politely, then tell them what you will do if they are over running – just in case. If you don't plan this in advance they will be shocked and you will be embarrassed when you have to interrupt them. Find out if they are staying after their talk, and so available for people to meet afterwards, or rushing off.
- Find out your house-keeping facts: where the toilets are, when and where breaks will be taken, what the fire alarm sounds like and what you should do if there is an alarm . . . and so on. Also check who will be your 'runner' during the sessions: it is very useful to have someone from the organisers, or a friend in the audience, close enough to be able to catch their eye if you want the air-conditioning turned up, or to bring forward the serving of lunch
- Set the stage (literally or figuratively, depending on the nature of the event): check that there are enough chairs for a panel session, that cables are tidied away, water and tissues are available, your table or seat is not obscuring the view of the screen, and you won't develop a torticollis looking up at it. At larger events, these things will be taken care of by the organisers, and a quick look around will reassure you. But it is definitely worth checking: it is you who will be stuck on the stage or at the front handling the problems! Put your clock or watch in place, or find a wall clock that is both right and working, and in your line of sight. Make sure you have a pen, paper and copy of the programme in front of you.

During the session

Whatever you do, don't drift! This is probably some of the hardest work you will do while appearing to sit quietly and serenely without a care in the world. You should:

- *take control*: be firm in welcoming people and telling them what you want them to do (like turn off their mobile phones). It is up to you to set the tone of the event:

upbeat, professional and in control

- *watch the time*: it is amazing how fast it can go, and even the most experienced speakers can get their timing wrong. Indicate as you have agreed when they are getting near the end of their time, and stop them, as arranged, if they over-run. Nothing makes an audience more nervous and restless than sessions running late
- *note a couple of key points, controversies or questions from the presentation*, in case you have to fill in because they finish early, or because the next speaker is delayed or equipment needs to be changed. Even if the timing is perfect, it is good to have a sentence prepared to link to the next speaker by saying something like 'Thank you for such a comprehensive overview of the regional situation on homelessness – now we welcome So and so, who will tell us about her service for homeless teenagers in X town'
- *keep an eye on the audience*: you can usually tell by watching faces and body language if people can't hear properly, or if they are hot, cold, bored or incensed. If there is clearly a general problem with the sound equipment or environmental factors, you can signal to your 'runner' to do something about it
- *support your speakers*: give the audience the lead by paying attention to the speaker, smiling and leading applause when appropriate, and laughing at their jokes. If the audience misbehaves – answering mobile phones, talking amongst themselves, leaving the hall – you will have to decide when to intervene to ask for attention to the speaker. Generally a quelling look from the chair will have the same effect without embarrassing the speaker, but you may need to say something, as neutrally as possible: 'I'm sorry to interrupt [speaker] – can I ask the audience for their attention to the speaker, please?'. If there is really bad behaviour – slow hand-clapping, heckling or jeering – you must intervene and say firmly that it is unacceptable. Such behaviour does happen, and I have known a chair let it continue unchecked. It was a very upsetting situation for everyone, including the majority of the audience
- *sit as still as you can while doing all of the above*: it distracts the audience and the speaker if you are bobbing and weaving in their peripheral vision
- if a speaker, or the whole session, finishes early, you can use your notes to sum up, but don't overdo it. Present it to the audience as an opportunity – to have a breath of fresh air, meet the speakers one-to-one or network with their neighbours – rather than a problem.

After the speaker

- Lead the applause.
- Start the questions if no-one else will.
- Indicate clearly to the speaker when they are free to leave the stage or podium.
- Be specific and clear in inviting other speakers to join you for a panel.
- Try to spread answering time evenly amongst panel speakers, so that one does not monopolise the time – but don't press them if a speaker does not want to contribute to a particular question.

- Don't plan a long summary or rousing speech at the end of the session – you will find people start to drift away anyway. Finish off warmly and succinctly, and let them go.

Expecting the unexpected

One of the things that keeps conference chairs on their toes is the knowledge that they have to deal with the unexpected, and the audience expects them to give a lead, whatever happens. Some of the unexpected scenarios that I have experienced at conferences and events include:

- three speakers cancelling on the day
- an air ambulance touching down outside the window, drowning out all attempts to communicate with the audience for 10 minutes
- a speaker who brought over 100 slides and expected to be allowed to discuss them all
- a speaker who finished halfway through her allotted time and invited the audience to 'share their experiences'
- an invasion by animal rights activists who had been chased out of another event elsewhere in the building.

There is no blueprint for what to do in these or other unexpected circumstances: it will depend on the time of day, the stage of the programme, the audience reaction, the significance of the event and so on. The key for the chair is to take charge, tell the audience clearly what decision has been taken in response to the situation and what they should do. And then manage the audience's reaction. Simple!

Things to do after a conference

It is vital to remember that the benefit you can get from a conference does not stop on the day – or it needn't if you do the associated 'homework'. Follow up contacts quickly, even if only to say 'it was good to meet you . . .' Then you will have less explaining to do if you want to get in touch a couple of months later. Sort through the information you have picked up, and the notes you made, and file the useful bits, so they don't simply sit in a pile with outdated papers. If you promised to send an idea, article or copy of something to a contact, do it quickly. If other people don't send you things you were expecting, follow them up.

PORTFOLIO POINTER

Summarise the key outcomes of the conference for you – new contacts made, article ideas offered, new information gained – and file them in your professional portfolio with the programme from the day to remind you of the date, venue and speakers.

CHECKLIST FOR ACTION

Have you:

- practised assessing conference programmes to pick out those that will meet specific development needs?
- planned how you will find a way to attend an extra conference in the next 12 months?
- put in an abstract to present a workshop session or poster?

CHAPTER 23

Writing letters

If you want to create an impact, write a letter. (Deb Lapthorne)

Writing letters sounds very simple: something we all do (or used to do, before email) routinely. Unfortunately, it is often done very badly, and a bad letter is worse than ineffective. It not only influences the opinion of the recipient about the letter writer, but also tempts him or her to assume the writer is representative of their whole profession. I have seen some embarrassingly poorly presented and written letters from practitioners in healthcare, sent to 'the very top' in the hope of influencing change, that painfully disguise the fact that the writer actually had a good point to make.

A good letter, however, is a powerful tool, when used sparingly and well. It can make an important point on a specific subject, in a way that is automatically recorded and retained. It can raise the profile of the writer, their organisation or their cause directly with a key person. And a series of well-crafted letters, with something genuine to say, can be used as a deliberate strategy to establish a reputation in a particular field, or with an important contact.

Always write to thank people when they have been helpful – make it personal, it means such a lot: everyone likes to be thanked. (Barbara Stuttle)

MIRROR MOMENT

Think about letters you have written – are there any you feel particularly proud of? Can you say why? Conversely, are there any that you really wish you hadn't sent? They might have been rambling, or very critical, or dashed off in the heat of the moment. The things that make you cringe about those letters are probably the best pointers towards a better letter in future.

Writing a good letter

> *Letters are best when short, to the point, courteous and well-presented. They say a lot about the writer and their organisation. If the contents convey a difficult or unwelcome message, there may be merit in putting in a warning call to the recipient first . . . especially if it is important to maintain a constructive relationship with the recipient.* (Sue Norman)

So what is the secret of a 'good' letter? Whether you are writing to your chief executive, your local council, a patient's group or a government minister, the rules are exactly the same. A good letter is simply one that:

- goes to the right person
- is sent at the right time
- delivers the right message
- is expressed in the right way.

Finding the right person

This is simple enough if you have information you want to give to a specific person (your resignation to your manager, or a comment on services to your GP): you write to them. It is less obvious if you want to give an opinion on the policies of the Government, the support you get from your professional organisation, or how a special interest group could revive its flagging fortunes. There is a regrettable tendency sometimes to 'go straight to the top'. Concerned about the future of physiotherapy services in London? – let's tackle the chair of the Royal Society. Local GPs being unhelpful about access to records? – report 'em to the local medical committee. Don't like the way care homes are inspected? – write to the Prime Minister. This approach is almost always unproductive, since the letter – particularly the intemperate or muddled letter – is unlikely ever to reach their desk, being winnowed out on the way by staff with a good eye for what the boss will want to know about.

Instead, find the right person to send it to: someone who will actually read it, and has the capacity to take action, or ensure that it is read and actioned at a higher level if necessary. Fortunately, in the age of the internet, it is relatively easy to find these people. Almost every organisation you might want to write to will have a website, and most (there are some inexplicable exceptions) will have a page of 'who's who' amongst the staff, in greater or lesser detail. Alternatively, you can follow the trail through department, directorate or specific service pages to the area you are interested in, and you may well find the name of the key person on that page. Sometimes there will be an opportunity to click on their name to email them (more about emailing rather than writing a letter on paper later), but in the meantime, this link can be useful if you don't find a postal address on the site, and need to email to ask for it.

The simple rule of thumb for identifying who you are looking for is that it should be the person closest to the action: there is a risk of looking (and feeling) very foolish if you fire off a letter to someone three steps away, who passes your letter back to the person at the first step, who immediately solves the problem, or answers the question, or explains the policy. So if you have a problem about permission for therapists to order X-rays in your trust, for example, start by identifying the key person in the radiology department to write to, rather than going straight to the medical director. If you want to let the Department of Health know about a new and successful project you have implemented in antenatal care, write to the professional advisor for midwifery, rather than a government minister. You may need or want to take it further, but everyone further along the line will expect you to have given your views to, or tried to resolve a problem with, the most appropriate person first.

If you are writing directly to a government minister, you can find the right one – with responsibility for the specific topic that concerns you – by looking on the department's website for details of each minister's portfolio.

PERSONAL DEVELOPMENT EXERCISE

Use the internet to find the names and email and postal addresses of the following people:

- the head of the school of nursing and midwifery at your nearest university
- the policy lead for cancer services in the Department of Health
- the allied health professionals lead in the NHS Alliance
- the lead on commissioning for older people's services in your local primary care trust
- the minister who currently holds responsibility for homelessness issues.

Going public

Finding the right person for a specific message is one approach. But what if you want to make a wider point through a more public statement? The commonest and easiest way to do this is by writing to a professional journal or a newspaper.

It is always easiest to write to one of the journals you read regularly yourself: you know their style, what kind of letters they publish, and what kind of readership they have. Journals, particularly the specialist ones, are often short of letters, and it is relatively easy to get into print this way. Having your name regularly on the letters page is a good way to raise your profile on a particular topic. And some journals publish letters not only giving opinions, or reacting to recent articles and editorials, but also reporting early findings of research, or asking for contacts in a particular field.

PORTFOLIO POINTER

Cut out and keep, or photocopy, letters you have published in journals: they are part of your professional development and often the first steps to more substantive publishing.

Writing more widely

It is worth considering writing letters to other journals – the ones you don't read regularly yourself – in order to make a point to colleagues outside of your own profession. There is a tendency for health professionals to be conservative – some might say parochial – in their reading and professional links, immersing themselves in increasingly specialist circles as their career develops. It certainly takes more effort to write to an unfamiliar journal, but it has potentially much greater impact. Like letters from patients in nursing journals, a letter from a therapist to a GP journal, or vice versa, is likely to catch the reader's eye.

There is some essential preparatory work before writing outside your usual area:

- look at a couple of issues of the journal to see what kind of letters they publish
- look at any aims or statement of purpose in the journal for an idea of their readership
- check for specific guidance on writing letters to the journal: some journals specify length, kind of content, the contact details they need from authors – some won't publish anonymous letters, but may be willing to withhold names in specific circumstances.

Whether writing a letter to a familiar or unfamiliar journal, it is also worth considering:

- whether your letter would have more impact if it came from more than one person: if so, look for appropriate joint signatories with relevant affiliations that will add weight to the letter
- whether your organisation has a policy about staff writing letters to journals, and if so, whether you should alert someone (your manager, or communications department) to the fact that you want to write to the journal, and seek permission, check the content with them, or simply send them a copy, as appropriate to the policy. Never send off a letter without checking and following the policy, in the hope that no-one will notice: you can be sure that someone will bring it to the attention of the appropriate authorities in your organisation!

Writing to the national newspapers

The same rules of preparation apply, but particularly the issue of following organisational policy. No organisation likes to find its name in the paper, particularly in the context of a comment, complaint or opinion that will be regarded as a statement of organisational views or policy. Communications people are experts and can help you make your letter better, or prevent you coming into conflict with managers.

If you believe that you have been unreasonably prevented from writing something, then there may be a bigger issue at stake. You need to consider whether your proposal was targeted at the wrong place – should you be writing to someone internally instead? If you believe your organisation is trying to cover up something that needs to be aired, then you need to look at your local 'whistleblowing' policy as well as talking to your manager (*see* Box 23.1). Don't tell yourself you can 'publish and be damned', in the old phrase: it sounds good, but is no comfort if you find yourself in a disciplinary hearing.

BOX 23.1 Need to know: 'whistleblowing'

- The Public Interest Disclosure Act 1998 came into force in July 1999. It protects 'whistleblowers' from reprisals, and secures compensation for people who have been victimised for revealing serious wrong-doing.
- Public Concern At Work is an independent authority on whistleblowing that provides free help to prospective whistleblowers, advising on the law and helping organisations to create a culture where it is safe and accepted for staff to report concerns. *See* www.pcaw.co.uk.

The right time to write

The timing of a letter can make all the difference to its effectiveness, and getting it right can be tricky. The following general rules seem obvious, but are frequently ignored:

- *if you are responding to an article or a letter in a weekly journal*: write within two days – a week later will be too late, as the next two editions will have been planned and the issue and correspondence will have moved on or been superseded. You can email these letters to the editor, so it should be possible to turn around your response in two days – providing you read the journal promptly when it arrives!
- *for journals with a longer lead time* – those published two weekly or monthly – still respond with a week, as they may be finalising pages well before the month end
- *responding to a consultation*: you genuinely have until the last day stated, as organisations are obliged to honour that: but look out for 'by midday on . . .' in the instructions, and allow plenty of time for 'snail mail'
- *commenting on government policy*: ministers will be away from Westminster for periods during the summer and at Christmas; avoid writing then, or in the run-up to a general election, when Parliament is technically dissolved and policies suspended. There may well be a new set of ministers, or a whole new party in government with a new set of policies, when it resumes.

> *Never send a letter or email in anger, hurt or frustration. Write it by all means but then destroy it. If in doubt, ask a close colleague what they think.*
> (ROSALYNDE LOWE)

One more point on timing: it is always a good idea, once you have drafted a letter, to put it aside for a short while, and then read it through again. It is surprising how often what felt like passion reads like petulance, and your heroic denunciation sounds more like a lunatic rant, on review. Give yourself a chance to put it right before you send it out into the big wide world.

The right message

Remember that people are very busy – layer your information, key messages first with further detail below – so they get the message quickly and can delve into more detail if they want to. (Judy Hargadon)

What is 'the right message' for your letter? I couldn't possibly say. The specific, headline message to be conveyed in your letter is whatever you want to say. But this section concerns the underlying messages, which are conveyed by the choice of words and tone of a letter. In my experience, it is fairly common for letters from practitioners to convey messages – often barely hidden – such as:

- 'I work with patients/clients, so my work is more important than yours'
- 'I don't understand your job but I think you're doing it badly'
- 'I hold you responsible for everything that's wrong with the health service'
- 'I could do your job better than you'.

Obviously there are few marks for courtesy to be gained from any letter that says this, even subliminally, to the reader. But more importantly from the writer's point of view, if you antagonise the reader – even if they are 'only' the person who passes letters on to the person who passes them on to the intended recipient – it may affect the way your letter is handled. Arrogant, irritating or insulting letters seem intrinsically less 'official' and therefore less urgent than well-written, objective ones. So always aim to be:

- positive rather than negative
- helpful rather than abusive
- offering solutions or suggestions, rather than criticism alone.

For example:

- *not good*: 'Therapists like us are totally frustrated by the ridiculous restrictions on the prescribing formulary'
- *good*: 'We are delighted that therapists are now able to prescribe, and we would like to suggest some additional medicines that could be added to the formulary to benefit our patients'
- *not good*: 'As a manager you obviously have no idea how difficult it is going to be for community dieticians to implement these changes'
- *good*: 'We would like to invite you to our monthly staff meeting so that you can meet the community team and hear about the way this change of trust policy will affect our work'.

It is important to realise that phrasing a letter positively, or objectively, does not mean that the message cannot clearly state an objection or criticism. It just does so in an acceptable way, rather than an antagonistic way.

Always use a heading or logo or stationery signature on every piece of communication, if you mean business. (Alexandra Lejeune)

The physical appearance of the letter also says something about its nature and importance. If you write to the prime minister on a grubby postcard or respond to a national consultation on a trust compliment slip (believe me, both have happened), then like it or not you are demonstrating a lack of professionalism that is read loud and clear at the other end, even as the information is being solemnly transcribed and handled. So, a few basic pointers:

- use A4 paper and business size envelopes, not anything more whacky than this
- coloured and lined paper doesn't qualify, unless you really need the lines
- for printing, use paper of at least 80 g in weight (normal copy paper); 100 g to make a really good impression
- handwritten is okay only if you have absolutely no alternative (surely not?), but many letters are scanned for electronic filing, and handwriting can be difficult to read in this form even if it is legible originally
- a plain font in a standard size (usually 12 point) is ideal.

When it comes to sending the letter, using the full, accurate address with the postcode, and the correct name and title of the recipient, is essential for a professional. Only 10 year olds can get away with writing to 'The Prime Minister, 10 Downing Street' and hoping for the best.

Expressing a letter in the right way

This is the real challenge of letter-writing: to convey the right message, and give the right underlying impression, in a way that makes the reader respond as you would want them to. Successfully getting the letter to the right person at the right time, on good paper with nice printing, is a waste of effort if the letter doesn't say what you want it to say when it gets there.

Many people in health and social care say they are better at verbal than non-verbal communication, at dealing with real people in their daily work, than writing things down. While essays and assignments are an accepted part of both undergraduate and postgraduate courses, many practitioners' day jobs do not involve a great deal of 'compositional' writing. So it is hardly surprising that skills get rusty and confidence fades.

MIRROR MOMENT

Be honest with yourself: how comfortable are you at expressing your views in writing? Does your heart sink at the thought – or do you quite enjoy putting words together? Now think about the last few months: when was the last time you wrote a formal letter – not counting clinical referrals or reports? Consider what you remember of the experience: what made it easier (quiet time, use of a template, drafting by hand before putting on computer?) and what made it harder (interruptions, your emotions, concern about the consequences?). These things are worth noting so that you can create the best possible circumstances for yourself next time you set out to write a letter.

Step by step

The good news is that the skill of putting together a good letter is soon revived (or learned), and it gets easier with regular practice. One helpful approach is to tackle it in stages:

- *stage one*: list the points you want to make
- *stage two*: decide on the framework for the letter
- *stage three*: insert the appropriate words in the frames
- *stage four*: check the draft against the points you listed at stage one: does it say what you wanted to say?

This may seem slower, because you are not launching into the letter immediately, but it does helps the letter to stay on track when you do begin to write it. It also means that you can write sections in any order. So, for example, you can write the paragraph with the suggestions or solutions that you are really enthusiastic about first – or the issue you are particularly exercised about – while it is fresh in your mind, and come back to the more prosaic first paragraph, which contains the reason for your writing and/or the link to the person receiving the letter, later.

An example without the stepped approach: a pharmacist is frustrated by the growing amount of *ad hoc* support she is giving to non-medical prescribers, and decides to write to the locality manager about it. Without planning, simply following her train of thought, the letter is likely to come out with a pattern something like this:

- complaint and annoyance
- implied slighting of nurses' and therapists' knowledge
- demand for change
- threat to withdraw help or complain elsewhere if this doesn't work.

This may make the pharmacist feel better for having spilled out her frustration, but is not very likely to result in a positive change or better interprofessional working. By followed the stepped approach, she would first sort out what messages she wants to give (stage one). These might be:

- the growing level of requests for advice from nurses and therapists about prescribing are interrupting my other work and causing a problem
- I do want to help but I need to have some control over when and how.

In stage two, the pharmacist decides the most effective and straightforward framework for the letter. This could be:

- *introduction*: who I am and why I'm writing
- *issue*: what the problem/purpose of the letter is

- *proposal*: options for what we could do about it
- *action*: what I suggest we do next
- *closing*: relationship building – positive words about the trust/other staff/services/ future.

Stage three is putting words into the framework. Just taking time to think about the messages and the outline of the letter may have dampened down the original emotions and result in a more neutral tone: but in case it hasn't, the main thing to watch at the writing stage is your use of language. Avoid exaggeratedly judgemental words (ridiculous, impossible, disgraceful) or embarrassingly effusive words (groundbreaking, amazing, fantastic) in formal letters. Aim in most cases for simple neutrality: *see* Table 23.1 for some examples.

TABLE 23.1 Using neutral language

Neutral	Emotive
I suggest that, or you could consider	Do this, you should
Changes, reducing	Cuts, slashing
Letter, circular, guidance	Directive, diktat
Staff, colleagues	The GPs, the care assistants

Stage four for the pharmacist is rereading the final draft of the letter to make sure that it still gives out her key messages clearly: she wants to help, but needs to do it differently.

PERSONAL DEVELOPMENT EXERCISE

Look at the letter in Box 23.2. It says something for the writer, but not in the clearest way that it could. Apply the tips above to redraft it – then look at Box 23.3 to see my suggestions.

BOX 23.2 A letter that could be improved

Dear Ms Evans

I am writing to inform you of the consequences on phlebotomists and other staff of your recent directives regarding the rearrangement of accommodation at the Brambleside Clinic which have cause major disruption to our services. It is impossible for us to see patients in the room in which we are now situated without access to our equipment stores that are now at the other end of the building. The district nurses' room is next door and when they are in a team meeting, this causes disruption to clinics in our room, particularly those of the audiologist, whose tests require a quiet and calm atmosphere. I notice that the trust has no trouble finding money for new furniture in the admin block, but there seems to be nothing available for the very reasonable plan put forward for a small extension to the clinic which would benefit patients and professionals, and improve services. I hope you will take time out of your busy schedule to do something about this.

(This letter is fictional but not exaggerated: I have read much worse.)

BOX 23.3 Alternative text for the letter

Dear Ms Evans

Accommodation for peripatetic staff at Brambleside Clinic

I am writing to ask for your help in re-organising the accommodation in this clinic to improve our services.

Since the recent change of rooms, we are working at some distance from our equipment supplies, and this is making it difficult to run our clinics effectively for our clients. Our new room is also noisy at times, making it unsuitable for audiology testing.

My colleagues and I would like to invite you to meet us at the clinic to look at the rooms available, and to discuss our ideas about reorganisation. I hope it may be possible to look again at the proposal for an extension to the clinic.

I look forward to seeing you.

Letters to journals

One time when you may be able – and encouraged – to break the rule of using neutral or positive language is in writing to the practitioner-type journals. Letters in these journals are less formal than in research journals, and more 'natural' language may be welcomed. You should though beware of being lured into trouble: some journals positively court controversial letters, extreme opinions and intemperate language, because it provokes a response from other readers, and sets up the letters page with lots of juicy copy for weeks. So don't expect the editor to counsel you to caution, to think of your career, or to consider the effect of your words on colleagues, managers and future employers. That is for you to do. You should always work on the assumption that the person you would least like to see your letter will be thumbing through the journal before you have the cellophane off your copy.

More on choosing words

In additional to careful use of words, there are some other very simple, but generally disregarded, tips for writing a good letter:

- use short sentences for impact
- use short words rather than long ones (use 'start' not 'commence', say 'I know' rather than 'I appreciate that . . .')

- use the active voice ('we produced these guidelines . . .') rather than the passive ('these guidelines were produced')
- avoid pomposity ('it has come to our attention . . .', 'in the unlikely event that . . .'), sarcasm and rhetorical questions ('have you any idea how . . .?')
- use minimal capital letters – for specific names of people, places and organisations only: not for 'trusts', 'social workers', 'patients' or 'residential care' in general
- remember that committees and organisations are singular entities, and verbs must match this: 'the association believes' while its members (plural) 'believe'; 'the committee intends . . .', but its members 'intend . . .'
- use regular new paragraphs to break up chunks of text
- don't ramble: say it and stop.

In summary, your letter should epitomise the 'four Ps': it should be polite, positive, purposeful and in plain English.

PERSONAL DEVELOPMENT EXERCISE

Gather some examples of letters that display the 'four Ps' – from journals, newspapers (the broadsheets are especially good for pithy, economical letters) and from work. Read them through a few times to get the feel of what makes them good.

Finishing off

One final point on putting the words into your letter: do check your facts. A very well-written letter that betrays a lack of knowledge you should be expected to have, or a disregard for the facts of the matter, will achieve nothing but damage to your credibility.

Having written the letter, set it aside for a day – then reread and check it against the messages you identified: does it say what you want it to say? Could it be more succinct, more objective, or clearer? Redraft if necessary, but not endlessly. At some point you need to stop and post it.

Email or 'snail mail'?

> *Do not use emails initially until you are absolutely confident that the recipient will appreciate the informality. I would attach a properly formulated letter to an email to initiate an idea then take it from there.*
> (MAUREEN WILLIAMS)

Who writes on real paper these days, you might ask? Isn't the whole world connected in cyberspace? Certainly almost all organisations are accessible via email and websites, from government departments to the smallest health-related charity and patient group, and most individuals within and outside the NHS have email addresses. The advantages of emailing over sending a 'hard copy' letter are obvious: it is instantaneous, doesn't require a printer or appropriate paper, a lengthy postal address, franking, stamps or the effort of dispatch. So there are times when an email is definitely the better way to send a message. It is most suitable when:

- your message is relatively short (anything that requires more than two paragraphs is difficult to read on screen)
- it is transient – relevant now, but not intended to be kept for posterity: email printouts are not an impressive sight in an official file
- you are having a regular dialogue with the same person, and/or
- you know the person you are corresponding with well
- you need to send the same message to a large number of people.

However, there are definitely times when a letter on paper is better. These are mainly:

- when you are writing formally with a view, response or point to make to a representative of an organisation
- when you are representing a group or organisation
- when you expect the correspondence to be kept and filed
- when you are making an impression on an important contact
- when you have more than a few lines' worth of things to say
- when you are targeting two or three people at most.

> *Solving disputes rarely works by email, it is often a symptom of avoiding conflict.* (Helen Mould)

There is of course a third way: if you have an electronic template with the headed paper of your organisation (and you are authorised to use it), or your home address if appropriate, you can write a 'proper' letter using the template, then email the document as an attachment to the recipient. Bingo! Speed *and* impact. However, unless you are also using an electronic signature, the letter will be unsigned. You may need to follow it up with a signed version.

> *It seems as if the whole world just uses email or sends texts but there are times when a formal letter is appropriate and knowing how to write such letters should not become a lost art. A formal letter can be sent as an email attachment!* (Joanna Parker)

Email hazards

If you are using email, you should always be aware of some major hazards unique to electronic communications that have caught out and damaged the reputations of many people. One is its speed of production and transmission. It is too easy to dash off an angry, indignant, insulting or indiscreet email and press 'send' before your higher brain functions kick in to stop you. We have all done it. There is no way back, only a further task, to delicately rebuild your relationship or reputation with the recipient.

The second hazard of email is the ease with which it can be forwarded to large numbers of people – so the impression you convey to the initial recipient can become your impact on another 10, 20 or 30 other people without you even knowing about it. No-one would photocopy a letter so many times and send it to lots of other people: but plenty of people forward emails to groups of people without a second thought.

Related to this is the hazard of accidentally including unintended recipients in your emails, giving them sight of inappropriate comments of information. Using 'reply to all' automatically means that comments you may only have intended for the sender are seen by other people too. The traditional advice 'If you can't be good, be careful' applies very well to the world of electronic communications.

> *Sometimes a reply sent to 'all' not only clogs the inboxes for people, but if you have not checked the circulation, you may find your reply goes to someone you would rather it did not!* (Judith Whittam)

Email groups

These can provide a very useful and rapid way of making contacts, sharing information, asking for help or advice, and commenting on news or developments. Always be aware however that they are being read by many people who do not know you, and will judge you on your contribution. Even 'closed' groups may have a moderator, and a wide variety of members with differing views. Open groups and chat rooms are visible to huge numbers of people. Consider what you say and how you say it, especially in this very informal atmosphere.

Writing a good email

There are many different views about email etiquette, and some organisations set out their own rules about how it should be used. As with writing letters, the key is to think of the underlying message that is read by the recipient along with your words. Unless it is going to someone you already know well, a misspelt and unpunctuated message, signed simply 'Joe Bloggs' or worse 'Joe', will suggest either carelessness or ignorance on your part, whatever the nature of the message. The familiarity we all have now with email communication seems to encourage this approach, even by people who are perfectly capable of writing coherently, and regardless of the importance of the message or seniority of the recipient. Some of the most irritating and unimpressive habits in emails include:

- no capital letters or punctuation
- disregard for spelling
- lack of complete sentences
- terse form of address, or no salutation at all
- demand for information with no courtesy please or thank you

- missing or first-name-only signatures with no clue as to who the writer is or where they are from.

Some of this may be simply a matter of taste, but it has an inevitable effect on the response of the recipient. A semi-anonymous, semi-literate few lines are much more easily ignored or deleted than a clearly stated and courteous request. *See* Box 23.4 for a comparison of the two.

> *Never type emails in capitals or in red.* (Judith Ellis)

BOX 23.4 Emailing a request for information

I have had many requests like this:

'hi could you sned me any information u have on mentoring and supervision thanks david'

I respond much better to requests like this:

'Dear Rosemary – I am a third year student nurse at Xshire University, preparing an assignment about mentoring and supervision for health professionals. I read on your website that you have recently published a report on this, and I would be grateful if you could send me a copy. Thank you. David Jones [address]'

Tips for effective emailing

> *If you're using email, don't copy the world in. I get very irritated with being copied in on everything – I expect people to have worked hard to solve something before they involve me.* (Alison Norman)

- Be descriptive in the subject line to help the recipient prioritise, find and file appropriately: e.g. not just 'presentation' but 'Clinical supervision workshop presentation, Social Work Today Conference, 18 April'.
- Avoid meaningless or frivolous headings in the subject line, like 'Hello' or 'Here we go again!': remember the original email may be responded to, passed on, copied to others and filed with that heading.
- Always use the recipient's name at the start rather than launch straight in to the message: with an appropriate salutation (hi, hello, dear).
- Copy in the minimum of people who need to know about the subject: don't use copying in as a bullying tactic.
- If forwarding an email, check whether you need to amend the subject line which may no longer be accurate
- Keep the text of the email short, simple and neutral: the speed and informality of email can tempt you to vent emotions and irritation in a way that will embarrass you afterwards. Unlike letters, emails cannot be intercepted and retrieved once sent.

- 'House-keep' your emails regularly. By creating folders to store those you need to keep, and deleting those you don't, you can keep your 'inbox' relatively clear, and you are less likely to overlook something you ought to respond to because it has disappeared off the bottom of the visible screen.

Exploiting the system

Some people already use all the technical tricks available to customise their computers. Some health professionals don't have regular enough access to a computer at work to have the luxury of doing so. But if at all possible, at work or at home, you should use the following both for your own convenience, and because it looks more professional to the person you are emailing:

- *set up an automatic signature on your emails*: give your name, job title, address, telephone and fax numbers, email address and website, if any. This saves you the trouble of writing it in when you remember that people might need it, and saves your recipient the trouble of having to email to ask you for an address to send things to. It also tells them where in the country you are, which can be useful for connecting you with local contacts or projects. Also, when emails 'bounce back', as they can do quite frequently for a variety of reasons, they can contact you by phone to let you know. You can set it up so that it is only used on external emails, so that brief messages to internal colleagues aren't accompanied by lengthy and unnecessary contact details
- if your organisation or group is advertising a conference, or if there is a specific message you want to disseminate – such as an imminent change of phone number, or new document available on your website – you can add a line or two beneath your contact details showing this
- *set up the system to notify you when an email is opened by the recipient*, if you are sending an important comment or response.

If you don't know how to do these set-ups, it is always worth asking a colleague, either professional or administrative – someone will know and people generally love to teach.

MIRROR MOMENT

What is your usual email style? Do you change it depending on who you are contacting? Think about ways that you could improve the impression given by your emails. Set up an automatic signature, if you haven't already, so that recipients have all the information they need to respond to you.

What happens after your letter arrives?

If your letter is reasonably written, and has been sent to the right person or journal, you should expect that something will happen as a result.

If it is written to an individual in a local or professional organisation, you could consider following up with a phone call in two to three weeks if you have not had a reply. This may be the start of a dialogue, and further involvement with the issue you have written about, which is why the impression created by your first contact is so important. Most organisations will have a quality standard for the time taken to acknowledge and/or reply to a contact: you could look this up on their website, or by phoning an appropriate department, before chasing a response.

If you have written to a government department, your letter is likely to be passed on to an official to prepare, or send, an answer. This will certainly be the case if you have written to a minister or senior official. They receive so much mail, it would be impossible for them to answer it themselves. For this reason there is little point copying your letter to lots of people in the department, since they will all end up on the desk of the official with the policy lead for the subject, or one of their team. You will receive an answer, however, and even if it is simply reiterating the very policy line that you wrote to comment about, you have at least registered your point and your interest in an effective manner. In fact, since ministers rather than officials decide policy, the latter are not empowered to change it, no matter how good a case you make! You should not expect an answer doing any more than explaining or elaborating on the policy line. This doesn't mean that it is not worth writing: your views will be lodged in the mind of someone working on the policy, and so potentially influence them in their future contribution to developing the policy – providing of course that you have targeted the right person. Sometimes professionals who have come to notice in this way are called upon later to join a group or give advice.

If you have written inviting a senior official or minister to visit a site, or speak at an event, your letter will be passed to an official to advise on whether the invitation should be accepted. You will receive an answer from a 'visits unit' or similar, though it may take some time. The same process applies if you have written to ask for a meeting, and in this case you should expect an answer from the diary secretary.

If you have written to a journal, you should of course scan the pages for your letter, and put it in your professional portfolio if it appears. Remember that all journals reserve the right to edit, so it may look a bit different. If you feel this has affected the message, you could write again to the editor asking to correct the false impression: journals are often good at printing your new letter in the next issue. If your letter provokes a response in the letters pages, you may be asked by the editor to read those letters in advance, and provide a response that can be published with them. You should always do so if asked. After all, you started it! Even if not asked, you may want to respond to further letters on the subject. This is a very good way of getting your name known and associated with a topic. In responding this way, the key things to remember are:

- keep follow-up letters short, otherwise they look defensive

- don't be scathing or dismissive, however silly the comments you are responding to
- if someone has pointed out a genuine mistake or omission in your letter, acknowledge it briefly and graciously.

If you have written in response to a consultation, your response may appear in full or in summary on the relevant organisation's website, unless you have specifically asked for it not to appear. Check this when sending your response in. You can use the website to check how other organisations and individuals responded to the same consultation. This may give you new ideas for further action on the subject – such as inviting like-minded responders to form a discussion group – or new people to contact and add to your network.

The Freedom of Information Act

This Act came into effect on 1 January 2005 (*see* Box 23.5). It requires all public bodies, including all NHS organisations, to make any information they hold available to anyone on request, with very few exceptions. This is worth remembering when you are writing to people in public bodies or responding to public consultations. At any time in the future, a journalist, patient or member of the public may ask for information held on a particular subject, and your letter may form part of the file. Contrary to popular belief, people's names are not routinely erased when papers are copied to be sent out in response to a request, nor is information assessed for relevance, importance or quality. If it forms part of the record on the subject requested, it will be sent out. This is not a reason to refrain from writing, just a good reason to be sure your letter wouldn't embarrass you if it should be passed on to a third party in future.

BOX 23.5 Need to know: The Freedom of Information Act

The Freedom of Information Act 2000 enables people to access information held by public authorities in two ways:

- *through publication schemes*: these make some information available to the public as a matter of routine, without a specific request being required
- *through a general right of access*: public authorities must respond to requests for information within 20 working days. This right came into force on 1 January 2005.

There are some exemptions to the information that must be provided by public authorities (such as NHS organisations, local authorities and government departments). These include, amongst others:

- information related to policy formulation, ministerial communications, law officers' advice (i.e. the legal advice given to ministers) and the operation of ministerial private offices
- information 'for the effective conduct of public affairs'

- **information reasonably accessible to the applicant by other means.**

Each of these exemptions is subject to its own guidance. See the website of the Information Commissioner's Office www.ico.gov.uk for full details.

Maybe the niceties of letter writing shouldn't matter in this day and age, but they do; and the more 'important' the organisation or individual you are writing to, the more 'old-fashioned' they are likely to be about these things. So it is worth playing the game, and making your letter as good as possible.

Email appears at first sight to provide an easier, more informal route to communicate with people you want to influence, but carries risks of its own. Taking it seriously and using it well and appropriately will greatly enhance your reputation and effectiveness.

Emails, letters . . . don't forget the phone! (SUZANNE HILTON)

CHECKLIST FOR ACTION

Have you:

- set up your email system with your 'signature' and contact details automatically included?
- found some good, succinct letters in newspapers or journals to learn from?
- written a letter to a journal?

CHAPTER 24

Writing papers for meetings

Keep asking yourself what you are hoping to achieve from the paper – and ensure that you stick to it. (LIZ PLASTOW)

If you want to influence a group of people, you are likely at some point to speak to them in a meeting. And in order to make your points, you will probably have a 'slot' on the agenda when they address your project, idea or point. For some meetings, this will automatically mean that you have to produce a paper to back your agenda item. For less formal meetings, you may not be asked to do so – but you may decide that it would be a good idea.

Why, you might wonder, would you volunteer for the extra work involved? Why not just turn up and state your case or give your report, let the other participants ask any questions they have, then off you go?

There are many good reasons for producing a paper for the meeting, even if you are not asked to:

- you can give more information than you could verbally
- you can give more complex information than you could give verbally
- information can be presented in more succinct ways, e.g. in a graph or a diagram
- you don't have to remember everything in the heat of the moment
- people will look at the paper as well as – or even instead of – looking at you, so reducing the glare of attention on you in the meeting
- the paper will make a more lasting impression, and be seen by more people than are present at the meeting to hear you speak
- there can be no dispute about what information you gave people as it is recorded in the paper.

This last can be important. If you are proposing a new way of working, and it is agreed at the meeting, no-one can say later 'You didn't say that this would double the care workers' mileage' if it was in your paper; or conversely, 'You told us the clients were in favour of this', if your paper made it clear that the three people you asked were in favour, but no full-scale survey had been carried out.

So, while it can be daunting to think of the five, ten or twenty people at the meeting scrutinising your writing, it is actually the lesser of two evils: they are less likely to be scrutinising you, and you are protecting yourself from future misunderstandings at the same time.

MIRROR MOMENT

How do you feel about your writing skills? Some people have no trouble dashing off a few paragraphs, but others agonise over choosing the 'right' words, or worry about their style, structure or spelling. If you are a worrier, and the idea of writing a paper every time you have something significant to discuss at a meeting fills you with despair, this chapter should help. The trick is to write to a formula, so that the choices you make are minimised and the task becomes easier and easier with repetition. If spelling, punctuation or use of English are real concerns to you, it would be worth doing some 'self-help' via a book, internet course or helpful friend: writing is so much a part of influence, and so many judgements are made on the basis of the emails, letters, papers and articles you produce (or fail to produce), that brushing up your writing skills is an essential part of your professional development.

Preparing a paper

The first rule is to let others do some of the work for you! So check if there is a standard format for papers for the meeting; look at any previous papers taken to the same meeting for a guide to length, style and format; ask the meeting organiser if there are any limits – such as one side of A4, no more than X words. Any guidance you can get on these factors will reduce your anxiety about whether your paper is going to be 'right', and make you more confident when you come to speak to the paper.

Secondly, stop to think about the purpose of the paper, which will guide the title, headings and content. Is it intended to update the meeting attendees on something they already know about? Or to introduce a new idea, project or proposal? Do you need a decision from them, or just comments? Are you reporting back, raising a new issue or asking for something specific? Once you are clear in your own mind what you want to happen as a result of your paper, and you have all the guidance or examples available on the sort of paper that is wanted, you are ready to plan.

PERSONAL DEVELOPMENT EXERCISE

Gather some examples of papers from meetings you have been to. Identify those that seem clearest and most helpful to you, and what makes them 'work'. These will be useful tips to apply to your own papers.

Planning the paper

> *Outline the aim of your paper and stick to it, don't wander off on tangents, no matter how interesting they may seem to you.* (LIZ PLASTOW)

The more descriptive the title, the better. It will help the people at the meeting if they can see clearly what your paper is about, and in the future, when the paper is filed away for posterity with the minutes of the meeting, it will be more easily retrievable by someone wanting to find it again. So, include all the key elements as succinctly as you can. For example, a paper called 'Midwife prescribing', could be about a whole range of things. Calling it either 'Proposal to introduce supplementary prescribing by midwives in the XX maternity unit', or 'Report of the evaluation of independent prescribing by community midwives in X locality' or 'Prediction of costs likely to be incurred by midwife supplementary prescribing in the X maternity unit' tells people much more. It helps to be explicit in the title about the status and nature of the paper: so calling it a report, a proposal, or an evaluation or feedback, is useful. So are qualifiers such as 'preliminary', 'final', 'internal' or 'confidential'. A fully descriptive title can head off some of the questions or objections that might be thrown at you if people misunderstood a vaguer title.

The format

> *Try to read previous papers that have been submitted. If there is a 'house style' you need to make sure that your paper is written in this way.* (LIZ PLASTOW)

A standard format really helps to take the work out of writing a paper. If you have the headings in mind, all you are doing is filling in the blanks. There is no 'right' format, of course, but the different lists of headings shown in Box 24.1 are two of the most useful options.

BOX 24.1 Useful formats for meeting papers

Option 1: Presenting an issue, problem or proposal

- *Summary*: if this was all they read, would they know what you wanted from them?
- *Issue*: summary facts and figures, outline of the situation.
- *Options*: what are the choices?
- *Recommendation*: what do you suggest they choose to do?
- *Actions/decisions*: what do they need to decide, or what do you intend to do next?

Option 2: Updating on a project or ongoing situation

- *Overview*: what the project/situation is all about, for someone who hasn't read previous papers/been at previous meetings; what you need from them.
- *Progress*: since the last update/meeting/paper – refer back to other papers rather than repeat.

- *Issues for discussion*: anything they need to take particular note of, or help you with.
- *Actions/decisions*: what do they need to decide (if anything), what are you going to do next?

The layout

Some simple guidelines will make your paper easy to read and use in the meeting, which will be greatly appreciated by the attendees, as well as making life easier for you:

- use subheadings and paragraph breaks to avoid dense blocks of text and help people find the interesting bits
- number paragraphs so that people can identify the bit they want to discuss in the meeting and others can easily find it (it's much easier to say 'paragraph 8' than 'the bottom of the second page just above the bullet points')
- keep the font to a reasonable size – preferably 12 point: if you are tempted to go smaller to fit it into the allowed length, or two sides of paper, cut words out instead
- minimise formatting – avoid italics, underlining, bold type, boxes etc which make it look fussy, denser on the page and harder to read.

Content

> *Make sure your paper has all the information needed for the decision – including the costs. It should answer all the questions you would ask if you were making the decision.* (Alison Norman)

Think minimal! Include only what must be said, and don't repeat facts unnecessarily. There is no need to rehearse government policy, local service configurations or geography, or the history of the situation, in a group where most people will (or should) know these things. If there is a longer or more complex section (and especially a table or graph) that you feel must be included, put it in an appendix at the end, so that it can be referred to, but does not get in the way of the main messages and decisions/actions required. Also, as this is a business document, there is usually no need to include academic-style referencing, however proud you are of your background research.

In choosing your words:

- *use plain English as much as possible*, and challenge yourself to find a shorter word whenever a long one comes to mind! There is a common tendency to adopt a more wordy style on paper than you would when speaking – try consciously to avoid this. So let work 'start' not 'commence', 'know' rather than 'be cognizant of' and report an 'idea' not a 'proposition'
- *keep sentences short*: it will be much easier to read – especially for those who are trying to read it in the meeting because they haven't done their homework!
- make the language appropriate for everyone present: so avoid uniprofessional jargon, or acronyms that are familiar to people from one organisation but will not

be known to others present, otherwise they will be made to feel outsiders

- *avoid value-laden language*: try to relay 'good news' or 'bad news' objectively, as some of the people in the meeting may view it differently and take offence. For example, saying in the paper that 'the council has been obstructive' will make local authority attendees or readers bristle. Saying 'the council has not agreed to support the plan' is equally factually correct, but less likely to cause offence
- *be absolutely clear when you want something from the attendees, by signposting it in the paper*. So you could finish the paper by saying: 'Does the steering group agree that (a) we should appoint a new project manager, and (b) the start date for the training should be put back to May?' This will help the chair to ensure that you get what you need from the meeting, rather than the discussion finishing inconclusively.

> *If there are financial implications, be honest and itemise amounts clearly. Be clear about what the outcomes of the project or work are, and ensure that they justify the cost.* (Liz Plastow)

Finishing the paper

You will need to finish the paper in time to send it to the meeting organiser to go out with the agenda. At all costs, avoid tabling a paper. It is unfair on the people attending the meeting, who then have to try to read the paper and listen to you simultaneously, or take your word for it that there are no hidden traps or pieces of bad news in the paper. At best they will think you are disorganised, at worst that you are deliberately trying to hide something. This applies particularly to papers involving figures, calculations or other complex content.

Before you consider it final, read through your paper and cut out some more words! This is always a good exercise: it is surprising how tight a piece of writing can be without losing the sense.

> *Always check your spelling. I recently saw a board paper that recommended that the organisation 'adopt' option 3, when what was intended was that we should 'adapt' option 3 – there is a world of difference!* (Alison Norman)

This is the point at which you might also want to mark the paper 'confidential', if appropriate, number the pages, and check that you have the date on it for future reference, as well as your name and the meeting it is intended for.

'Speaking to' your paper

> *When presenting your paper, be enthusiastic and optimistic. Really try to sell yourself and your paper. Dress appropriately for the audience and abide by the etiquette of the meeting, referring back to the chair as appropriate.*

If you are not enthusiastic, you cannot expect your audience to be.
(Liz Plastow)

When your agenda item is introduced, you will usually be invited to 'speak to' your paper, or 'tell us about it', or something similar. This is a chance to draw attention to the key issues – not rehearse the whole paper. Remember:

- don't read out any portion of the paper
- start by summarising the summary
- point out any particularly interesting, relevant or important points, or things that have changed since you wrote the paper (having highlighted them on your copy earlier so that you can be confident about paragraph numbers)
- be clear if you are inviting comment or debate from members present at any point
- ask very clearly for any key decisions: 'which option do you prefer?', 'do you agree that . . .?', 'what should I tell the regional group?'

PERSONAL DEVELOPMENT EXERCISE

Practise writing short papers for meetings, even if you are not asked for them – for example, for a team meeting. Use them as a way of collecting your thoughts concisely, and planning what you will say or ask for at the meeting. When you are confident about doing them, start to offer to write a paper on a relevant topic for other meetings you attend.

Why writing matters

If your aim is to influence change, and reach outside your own organisation to regional or national groups or leaders, then you will need to be good at written communication. Writing – whether papers, letters or emails – will be seen by many more people than will ever meet you in person or hear you speak. Practising good, succinct writing for meeting papers will benefit your other writing, and greatly improve your reach and your influence.

CHECKLIST FOR ACTION

Have you:

- identified some examples of 'good' meeting papers you can learn from?
- written some practice papers for meetings you go to?

CHAPTER 25

Influencing policy

Choose your battles carefully, they must be worth the fight and possible to win. (HELEN MOULD)

While there are different forms of 'policies' in many organisations, this chapter focuses on influencing government policy related to health and social care. People generally have one of three reactions to this idea: 'it can't be done'; 'I'd like to influence policy but don't know how to go about it'; and 'I know where they're going wrong and I emailed the Prime Minister yesterday'.

To answer these in order:

- you can exert some influence over the development of health policies, if you are prepared to do the necessary work and put in the effort, preferably working collectively with others. This doesn't mean that your idea, solution or good practice is likely to be adopted wholesale – there are too many other influences on the policy process for that. But your contribution can help to steer the ship in a better direction
- how to go about it is the substance of this chapter – once you have done the background work of making yourself aware of the policy area you want to influence, as described in Chapter 13.
- and yes, there are people who write directly to the Prime Minister with their views on policy – but there are better ways of ensuring that your contribution is read, valued and effective. This chapter explains how it can be done, and some ways you can make your contribution.

Get a constituency – either of ideas or people – so you are representing the views of a network or people at work, not just yourself. (ALISON NORMAN)

Approaches to influence

To influence nationally it has to be done through a structure or organisation, like a union. Local activism can help – but remember political parties come and go. (ALISON NORMAN)

There are three approaches to having a say on policy, each of which will be appropriate to different people in different circumstances at different times:

General approach

This involves writing articles and opinion pieces about your subject for the relevant professional press; speaking at conferences; networking with a wide range of other people involved in the same field; and contributing to professional debates via letters pages or at local, regional or national meetings. Other chapters in this section give specific advice on these activities. You may not be aware of any policy makers or officials hearing or reading what you are saying. But these people are also reading, networking, attending conferences and listening to the professional debate. The views, responses and attitudes put into the public arena by you and others through these activities will form part of their thinking. This is the most indirect route to influence – but very genuine. Do not underestimate the credence given to frontline health and social services workers, and their experiences. And sometimes influencing in this way leads to more direct routes. I have certainly invited people whose articles I have read, presentations I have attended and opinions I have heard, to join policy advisory groups, or to attend meetings with ministers. *See* Box 25.1 'need to know' for more about 'policy makers'.

BOX 25.1 Need to know: who are the policy makers?

The officials in government departments who work on specific policies are often thought of as the policy makers. It is important to remember that their role is to advise ministers on policy, and in doing so they have great influence over the way policy develops – but the final policy decisions lie with ministers.

A wide range of other people are involved in influencing, shaping and developing policy, and are worth thinking of when you are looking to influence policy. They include:

- senior post holders in planning and commissioning organisations such as health and local authorities, who meet regularly with senior policy officials
- professional leaders such as heads (or heads of health) of trade union and professional organisations, who are often consulted throughout the policy process and invited onto advisory groups
- clinical directors and heads of professions within the Department of Health
- leaders of major organisations representing patients and carers, who are often invited onto reference groups
- MPs and peers in the House of Lords who may initiate or contribute to debates on relevant issues, and help or hinder the passage of legislation.

Focused approach

> *Have the confidence to contact the policy leaders – know that they want contact.* (Judith Ellis)

This is a rather more organised attempt to influence policy. It involves joining specific interest or lobbying groups, responding to public or stakeholder consultations on 'your' topic, and targeting information, good practice examples or offers of help to specific policy contacts. This approach depends on building good relationships, good working practices and a good reputation, to avoid simply becoming a thorn in the side of policy officials (*see* other chapters in this section for effective ways of operating in groups, writing letters, influencing in meetings, etc).

> *Work out what the policy makers may want – their perspective.* (Fran Woodard)

Specific approach

> *One of the most important factors in developing my career was being involved at national level with my professional body. It gave me great insight into national issues and taught me how to be influential in meetings.* (Sandra Mellors)

There will be times when you feel strongly about the direction of policy, or a specific policy proposal, and want to take the most direct approach to influencing the proposal or its implementation. This is when formal letters to officials, MPs or ministers may be appropriate, or you may want to organise a group response, request a meeting with a policy lead, or invite an official or minister to visit your service or organisation.

Each of these approaches may be the right one in different circumstances. Whichever approach you choose, the key is to know how to go about it in a way that will enhance, not damage, your reputation, and be most successful in influencing the policy you want to address.

> Top tip: *develop political savvy. Gain insight, learn good timing and the use of trade-offs.* (Fran Woodard)

MIRROR MOMENT

Which of these approaches feels instinctively like the one for you at the moment? Is there something so urgent and important that you want to try the specific approach – or are you thinking of moving from the general to a more focused approach on a specific topic? If you haven't yet taken on any of the activities that constitute a general approach, it would be wise to try some of these before going for something specific. They build your confidence in your self, your experience and your views, as well as giving you a reputation to build on when you start to make contact with policy makers.

The policy process

> *Find out who or what group is responsible for the policy and get to know the purpose and 'direction of travel'. Search out ways of conveying your well-evidenced argument to them if you can't do so face to face.* (SUE NORMAN)

Before looking at some specific techniques, it is worth stepping back to take an overview of the policy-making process, and to look for opportunities to intervene and influence.

There is not really a logical, sequential pattern to the way that health policies are developed, but unpicking the bundle of activities involved generally exposes the following steps, even if in real life they rarely occur in a neat ordered sequence:

- *the idea*: e.g. centralise specialist expertise in 'hub' centres, or treat more people at home, or do something about the rise in obesity. There are many sources for these ideas. They may arise from new research findings or statistics, from a series of news reports, from party ideology, ideas from abroad, pressure from interest groups, the advice of key committees or simply from someone in government seeing or experiencing an example of good or bad practice. Individual healthcare workers, groups or professional organisations can bring ideas, examples of innovative practice, information, research and patient needs to the attention of policy makers through letters, articles, group representations and contributions at conferences
- *working up the idea internally*: civil servants produce submissions to ministers setting out ways in which the idea could be turned into a working policy, including pros and cons, costs and impacts, likely reaction from different groups, and so on. They will often look for 'experts' or experienced professionals to contribute to reference groups to guide thinking and bring a voice from the frontline. This is where building your expertise and profile through writing articles, speaking at conferences and hosting site visits or study days, reaps benefits by raising your profile and making you much more likely to be invited
- *consultation*: this may be formal, with a written document published for the public or specific stakeholders to respond to; or informal, involving floating the ideas at meetings, in conference speeches or individually to key groups or individuals, to see how they are received. Responding to a consultation is a simple and effective way to engage with the policy-making process
- *decisions*: any significant policy decisions are made finally by ministers, not officials, once advice has been given, consultation responses reviewed and any further information or options explored. However, many of the details and plans for implementation will be put together by officials, so having them in your network and offering constructive ideas to them can be genuinely influential
- *announcement*: decisions on new policies and key milestones in existing work may be announced in a speech by a minister or senior official, or set out in a press release, or made available in policy documents on the department's website – depending on the degree of attention the department wants them to attract. The

responses to public or stakeholder consultations are often posted on the relevant department or agency's website. These can be used to check how far the decisions taken reflect the responses received

- *communication*: throughout the process there are announcements, statements and publications that explain what is planned, and why, how it should be implemented and how it will affect local services and local people. It is a good idea to read the original policy documents from the department's website in order to get the full story. Checking for 'what's new' and 'press releases' helps keep you up to date on the progress of a policy. Also look out for articles in journals by officials. *See* Chapter 13 for more about how to stay aware of policy
- *legislation*: if the policy requires new legislation to either allow, or require, organisations, professionals or relevant agencies to implement the policy, this is an enormously detailed and time-consuming process. As well as completing the drafting of the legislation, a slot has to be found in the legislative timetable for it to go through lengthy parliamentary processes. *See* Box 25.2 for more about different forms of legislation. It is useful to know something of the terminology and processes to avoid making unrealistic demands of policy makers, and to impress them with your attention to detail!
- *implementation*: this now generally happens at the level of individual NHS and social care organisations, with guidance and advice from strategic health authorities or local authorities, rather than being 'run' by a regional tier or organisation. This provides further opportunities, as the way that a policy is put into practice locally is often open to local influence. Some policies change greatly at this stage, becoming practically tailored to provide more benefit to the client group, so this is not an insignificant contribution to make. It is worth trying to encourage your organisation, professional group or team to volunteer to be a test site (or 'pathfinder', 'beacon', 'spearhead' or whatever the current term happens to be) for new ideas: early implementers (there's another one) are often very influential, having privileged access to policy makers and sometimes ministers, and a chance to feedback their real experience and modify or develop the policy. This is one of the clearest examples of how frontline staff help to shape policy
- *evaluation*: this final step can feed in to the 'ideas' that keep the policy process evolving and developing. How well modern matrons, new arrangements for inspection of care premises, or changes to invalidity benefit achieved their objectives, according to independent research evaluating them, affects future decisions about taking related developments forward.

So the opportunities to influence policy exist at every stage, from the original idea to development and implementation. But how should you do it?

BOX 25.2 Need to know: understanding legislation

Some key terms that are often heard when discussing health and social care policy and potential changes to legislation are worth understanding and using correctly.

- *Bill*: a document setting out a proposed new law, or amendment to existing law, for consideration by Parliament.
- *Public bill*: one that will have general application if it becomes law; may be proposed by the government, or by a specific MP, when they are known as private members' bills (the first bill to introduce nurse prescribing was a private members' bill).
- *Private bill*: one that will apply only to a specified group e.g. people in one part of country, if its proposals become law; promoted by a particular group or organisation, not by the government or an MP (though it does require a parliamentary sponsor).
- *Act*: the legislation resulting from a bill having successfully completed its passage through both Houses of Parliament (Commons and Lords) and received the Royal Assent from the monarch.
- *Primary legislation*: Acts of Parliament; provide the overall framework of law on their topic.
- *Secondary legislation*: delegated legislation made under a 'parent' Act of Parliament; contain more detail than primary legislation, and can be amended without the same degree of parliamentary scrutiny – and in some cases, none. It includes statutory instruments (SIs), orders and regulations.

Some specific actions

> *One of the most important factors in developing my career was realising that my comments on policy are listened to – but you have to comment in the first place.* (Helen McCloughry)

Most of the general and focused approaches described above have been covered in other chapters: writing letters and articles, making presentations, influencing in meetings, and using special interest groups. Below are a number of other, more specific techniques – often employed inappropriately and so ineffectively – that could be used when there is a specific issue you feel you must respond to.

> *It is about making sure you know 'who' to talk to, who are the people with influence.* (Monica Fletcher)

Writing to your MP

> *Remember that things which are obvious to you may not be to others, so engage in consultations whenever possible.* (Helen Mould)

This could be appropriate where the issue of concern is local, or if your MP has a particular interest in the health or social care issue you wish to raise – which you could find out from his/her website. It is not generally appropriate to write to them on national policy matters. In putting the letter together, follow the guidance for writing letters in Chapter 23. Keep the language simple and the content short, objective and accurate. State the issue clearly, and provide something constructive: if not a proposed solution, a clear suggestion for what would help the situation. You can find your local MP's constituency address from their website, or, when Parliament is sitting, write to them at the House of Commons.

Your MP may decide to write to the Secretary of State or a minister in a relevant department, enclosing your letter, particularly if he has had several similar letters from constituents. In this case, the minister will respond to the MP, and your MP may respond to you to let you know what that response said. This process often takes many weeks, as the letter will be sent out from the minister's office to policy officials to provide background information, advice and a draft response. For responses to MPs, this will be returned to the minister's office for reading and signature before dispatch.

Writing directly to a minister

This can be appropriate (usually for a group or organisation rather than an individual) on national policy issues, rather than local implementation concerns, but is a tool to be used sparingly. Contrary to belief, inundating a minister with lots of letters often has less impact than a single letter – particularly when the many letters are on the same subject and/or copied to other ministers or the Prime Minister. This does not attract any more attention, as they will all be sent out as a linked set to the same officials for background, advice and a draft response. All it achieves is to look amateur and intemperate to those officials – who are exactly those you need to be impressing because they work on your area of interest!

If you are writing to a minister, follow the usual rules for a good letter. Target it accurately, by checking which minister speaks, makes announcements or is named in public policy documents on the subject you are writing about. Be as constructive as you can, even if you are writing with deep concern: everyone responds better to offers of help than to criticism.

When your letter arrives in the minister's private office, it will be dispatched to the relevant person in their department for advice and a draft response, just like an MP's letter. But in the case of letters to ministers, some will be marked for response by an official – in which case you will get a letter directly from the policy official – and only a few will be marked for return to the private office for signature by the minister. This is not an insult, just a way of handling enormous amounts of post. Bear in mind that minister's replies are drafted for them, and the officials' role is to promote and defend the policies of the government of the day – so you are likely to receive the same response to your letter, whoever signs it.

Postcard campaigns

These are often organised by unions to send a 'blitz' of paper in to ministers' offices, in order to indicate the strength of feeling amongst their members. If you use this method, bear in mind that it will not link you personally to the campaign. It may work to exert the pressure of numbers, but there are more effective ways of you personally influencing policy.

Invitations to ministers/senior officials

If you think you have a good example of innovative working, excellent care for patients or clients, or significant new research findings, you may want to invite a government minister or senior official – a head of profession, or department lead on your subject – to a site visit or to speak at an event, in order to influence them. Again, this is a tool to be used sparingly, as they may accept, and you want to be sure that you have something sufficiently substantial, tested and successful to say or demonstrate. However, visits to sites doing innovative things have been known to result in rapid national uptake into policy, so they can be a very effective way to influence.

Clearly, issuing such an invitation is normally a matter for the most senior person in your organisation. But if you are chair or secretary of a national group, or you work independently and lead your own organisation, you may be that person. Before making the invitation, you should consider the impact of a visit or speech by a minister. It will take up a lot of time, require complex and detailed arrangements and liaison with his/her office, and overshadow other speakers, events or pieces of work. You will have no control over what the minister says, the purpose to which the visit is put, or how it is reported. There will be greatly increased media interest, and the focus will be on what the minister says or announces, rather than the rest of the programme. It is also possible that the visit or attendance will be cancelled at short notice – even on the day – no matter how much notice you have given, due to competing demands from parliamentary or party business. It is a very good idea to have a 'plan B': either an alternative speaker who has agreed to step in at short notice; or a rescheduled programme that fills the gap with some other planned and relevant activity. Either is infinitely preferable to 30 minutes of nothing!

Inviting a minister is undoubtedly a risky strategy – inviting senior officials slightly less so, but not dissimilar – but if you do embark on it, the following should help you:

- make the invitation in a letter, giving full details of the event (audience, purpose, numbers, venue, programme, other speakers) or potential visit (what is new/ different, where it is, what can be seen). Make clear why the minister or official would want to come: does it give them a platform to speak to key people, showcase the kind of work they have been advocating, benefit groups they have been championing, or what? It is good to give several months' notice of an event, although ministers' schedules can be very fluid and they may accept at short notice if they can see the benefits to them
- the invitation will go to officials for advice on acceptance – another reason to have built a good reputation with relevant policy makers, or at least in the professional press and conference circuit. You may be asked to provide more details at this stage – needless to say, you should respond very promptly, helpfully and politely. If you then receive a letter declining the invitation, accept it gracefully. Many such invitations come in, ministers have genuinely busy lives, and it is not a

snub to be turned down. You will have done your reputation, and that of your organisation, colleagues and project, no harm if you have handled the whole process well

- if the invitation is accepted – stand by to be told what to do by the minister's office. They are likely to want much more detailed information and briefing, and to need almost undivided attention for the final few days as well as on the day. They may want to change the length of time allocated to the minister, the positioning of the slot in the programme, or the nature of the minister's contribution. For example, they may want him/her to have a question and answer slot, or to be 'present' via videolink from somewhere else. It is essential to take their requests seriously, respond quickly and accurately, and provide what they ask for. This is not the time to decide you are too busy, or your other work comes first. If you don't have the capacity to handle the visit, don't ask for it. Once it is happening, enlist as much help as you can, and let the private office staff guide you
- quite often, an invitation to a minister or senior official results in the offer of an alternative person to attend the visit or speak at the conference: usually a relevant department official. This is a great opportunity to influence them on a one-to-one basis, and should be accepted. They will be a lot less trouble than a minister in terms of security and impact on your event or organisation, but bring a lot of valuable inside knowledge. Do not treat them as a poor substitute, even if you know your audience will be disappointed.

Timing

The timing of letters, invitations and campaigns can be affected by the electoral cycle, and is worth considering. For example:

- as soon as a general election is called, Parliament is officially dissolved and the policies of the current government are suspended. This means that civil servants and officials cannot speak about these policies, or develop them further. This period is often referred to as election 'purdah'. Clearly it is not a good time to write a letter or invite an official to a meeting. If you have an official or minister booked to speak at an event, they are very likely to cancel
- in the year running up to an expected election – but before it has been called – the government will be particularly concerned with demonstrating the success of its policies, and the benefits they have brought to both patients and the public, and healthcare workers. This is a good time to bring forward examples of good practice or innovation, but not an effective time to propose major changes, or point out significant flaws. If you are starting to plan an event or campaign during this time, remember the potential for the election to disrupt your plans
- immediately after an election is a good time to pinpoint how your project, innovation, issue or concern can be targeted to fit with the new government's policies and priorities, as these will have been made explicit in the party's manifesto during the election campaign. Remember that even if the same party is returned to Parliament, there may well be a reshuffle of key personnel: check

the website of the government department most relevant to your work to see who are the responsible ministers and policy leads post-election.

Meetings with ministers

> *Find out who the policy makers are and meet with them to discuss your ideas. Be proactive in implementation, you will find policy makers then ask you for your views.* (Barbara Stuttle)

Suppose all your networking, writing, speaking and innovating has paid off, you are known to policy makers as someone who knows what they are talking about and has useful things to say – then you could find yourself invited to meet one of the government ministers to talk to them about your area of practice, usually as one of a small group. This is of course a key opportunity to influence: but also a daunting prospect even for the most senior and confident of people. It is useful to have an idea of what to expect and how to be most effective in the meeting.

Arrangements for the meeting

These will be made by the minister's private office. You will probably have no more than 45 minutes, and possibly less. This may seem very little, if you are travelling a long way for the meeting, but that is how it is: the minister will have many such meetings back-to-back on the day. Be prepared for the time to be altered, possibly at short notice, for the minister to be running late, and sometimes for the meeting to be cancelled at short notice. It is frustrating, but unavoidable, and the private office staff will try to ensure that you know about it as early as possible. For this reason it is a good idea to give them a mobile number as a contact for you. If you are going to be out of your workplace on the day before the meeting, or setting off early to make the journey, make sure someone is looking out for any message or email about changes, and will pass it on to you immediately. On the day, arrive in good time, but expect to wait. You may be met by an official from the department who will tell you something about the format or nature of the meeting. If they give hints about the best way to approach a subject, or a point to avoid, it is worth taking note.

Preparing for the meeting

> *If you believe in what you are saying, make it sound like you do! Talk with authority, clarity and a firm belief that the knowledge you are imparting is right.* (Judith Whittam)

Make sure you know why you have been invited, who suggested your name and what is expected of you. Find out from the person who sent the invitation whether you are there to represent your piece of work, your profession's opinions, your organisation or special interest group, or another perspective. Then make sure you have the necessary information, briefing and permission to do so. Facts and figures, examples of practice and stories from 'the frontline' are valuable contributions, and worth jotting down on a crib sheet as a reminder. Look up the minister on the department's website so that you know what areas of policy they are responsible for, and what their background is: this can save you the embarrassment of talking about something they are not interested in, or telling them things they already know very well.

In the meeting

> *Do not get personal but use anecdotal evidence sparingly and only if you have to. Much better to evidence your arguments with properly thought-out angle and direction.* (MAUREEN WILLIAMS)

With time being short, and a group of people wanting to be heard, you should try to make sure that your contributions are short, clear and to the point. Use your information selectively rather than trying to give it all, and concentrate on making two or three key points. Writing these down in advance is useful. Time is of the essence, so be ruthless with yourself, discarding the quantity of information you would like to give in favour of the quality of your key points.

> *Personal behaviour is important – be prepared to compromise, listen and negotiate, check your facts, be polite, and be prepared to be part of the team.* (BARBARA STUTTLE)

Other people

There is likely to be both a policy official and a member of the private office staff in the meeting, taking notes. They generally expect to be ignored, so focus your contributions on the minister – while noting the name of the policy official for later contact, if you don't already know it. If you are in a group of people, resist the urge to compete to contribute, which looks unprofessional. Don't repeat a point already made, or simply add another anecdote to theirs: try to move the discussion forward, or make a new point following on. Don't expect to get new information from the meeting, or challenge the minister to tell you what is planned next in your area of interest – they are unlikely to crack under your interrogation! Instead use the opportunity to raise the professional or service issues that should inform the next policy steps.

> *If challenging a policy, provide positive alternatives or amendments.* (JUDITH ELLIS)

End of the meeting

With such busy calendars and short meeting slots, it is essential to private office officials that their minister finishes meetings on time. Expect the meeting to be cut off at the fixed time, however interesting or important the discussion, and to be hustled out of the room. This is not a reflection on you, the group, or indicative of a failure to engage the minister's interest: just practicality.

Afterwards

You could email the policy official who was at the meeting, or the one who arranged for you to be there, and thank them for the opportunity. At the same time, you could provide the other material you had ready for the meeting but weren't able to use, giving them more reasons to stay in touch with you.

Being effective in influencing policy

To summarise, the factors that will make you effective at influencing policy are the simple ones – but all too often overlooked. They are:

- a professional approach
- courtesy in communication
- background knowledge and awareness of the subject
- lucidity and brevity in communications
- constructive suggestions
- prompt responses to requests for information
- understanding the system and its constraints
- respect for other people's expertise and priorities
- robustness and persistence.

Common mistakes that undermine attempts to influence policy are:

- copying in lots of people to letters or emails
- emotional and insulting language
- criticism without constructive suggestions
- being uninformed and unaware of existing policy
- expecting your solution or suggestion to be adopted unchanged
- blaming the wrong people for perceived faults with the policy.

> *A common mistake is being persistently negative with few, if any, alternative suggestions.* (Sue Norman)

It would be nice to say that these behaviours were rare in people who make the effort to try to influence policy on health or social care – but they are not. The good news is that this makes the people who do go about it in a more professional way stand out and be appreciated by beleaguered policy makers!

> *You'll know you've succeeded when your ideas are presented as the original idea of the policy maker!* (Rosalynde Lowe)

CHECKLIST FOR ACTION

Have you:

- looked up the lead ministers and policy officials for your area of interest on the relevant department's website?
- decided what kind of approach to influencing policy is appropriate to you at the moment?
- undertaken some of the 'general' influencing activities described at the beginning of the section?

SECTION 4

Being visible

CHAPTER 26

Coping with the consequences

One of the commonest mistakes is to believe all the negative comments – then hibernate. (Barbara Stuttle)

Some people try to gain influence in the NHS or social services solely because they want to improve care or services for the people who use them. Others do it because they want to build a high-flying career, become a respected expert in their field, or gain status and a national reputation. Most people probably combine some element of both these motives, whatever they say on their job applications.

No matter what the motivation, it is a fact that doing the work and developing the profile that allows you to have influence brings with it some inevitable consequences. It is as well to anticipate, accept and deal with these. This chapter looks at how you can prepare for, and handle, some of the consequences of your success in gaining awareness and influence.

The consequences of you gaining a profile and influence will be felt by:

- you and your family
- the people you work with and for
- others in the service and profession whom you don't know.

Consequences for you and your family

If you have worked through the sort of exercises described in early sections of this book, or been doing these kinds of activities before, you will know that they always take up some of your own time. It is a fallacy to think that you can develop the sort of awareness you need, doing the reading, researching, emailing, writing and networking, in 'work time'. Investing some of your own time at evenings and weekends, days off and holidays, is part of the deal. It does not all have to be done in your own time: the division between work and professional outside activities is not that sharp, and every meeting, client contact and paper at work is an opportunity to learn, or to develop useful skills for influence. But some of your own time will be needed. It may be time on the internet, or time spent reading journals, writing articles, making an evening phone call, or travelling back from network group meetings later in the day.

The consequences of this will depend on each individual's circumstances: who else is competing for that time, how tolerant they are of your 'time out', how much help you have with other home activities. Some people find that their families are resentful of their 'extracurricular' activities, which can cause tensions in the most tolerant of households when there are other, competing demands on time. To minimise problems:

- be open with your partner/family about what you are doing and why: if they think you are doing unpaid overtime for work they may resent it; but if they know you are pursuing something because you are interested, or because it is going to help you get your next job, they may be much more tolerant
- use as much 'intermediate' time as possible for these extra activities – time on a train, in a waiting room, doing housework or waiting for the second half of the match to start can be used for reading articles, planning a presentation, or thinking about how to word an important letter. This is time you then don't have to spend hidden away in a study, or behind a journal, when people want your attention
- share your successes with the family, don't save them for your CV: when all your extra effort results in an invitation to an important meeting, or your article is published, or your comments get a positive response from a key individual, let your family share the satisfaction and get a positive reward for enabling you to put that effort in
- make sure you keep and protect some genuine 'down time' – however ambitious, driven or enthusiastic for change you are, you will be more effective if you are adequately fed, rested and rounded! You personally need to ensure that there are times outside of work when you are *not* thinking about your next article or email to the policy lead. Other interests, time spent with the partner or family, and physical activities help to do this. Equally, those around you will be happier if they know there are always times (not just on formal family holidays) when they have your undivided attention and presence.

It is important not to misinterpret the thrust of this book: it definitely does not advocate spending every waking minute on the pursuit of awareness and influence!

Consequences at work

> TOP TIP: *understand how you are perceived, your standing and reputation.*
> (FRAN WOODARD)

Getting involved in the extra activities that develop awareness and build influence can have consequences in your 'day job' as well. It is as well to be sensitive to the views of your colleagues and managers, to anticipate problems before they arise. People may resent having to cover when you go to meetings or network groups, or having to change their way of working because you are putting new knowledge into practice. They may feel that you are trying to 'get ahead' at their expense, or that you see yourself as better than them – or indeed better than you are! Sometimes colleagues will feel they are carrying your work because 'you are never there'. Of course, there are teams and workplaces where such issues never arise – but in my experience, these reactions are not uncommon and can be very hard to handle. Some tactics to handle these reactions include:

- *keeping colleagues informed*: let them know where you are going, who you are talking to or what is the purpose of a meeting, so that they are aware of the reasons for your absence
- *involving people*: ask for their ideas, views and suggestions, and let them see that their contribution is valued and taken into account
- *feedback*: let people know what was decided at a meeting, show them your article, or the response to your letter. If you can't speak to people personally, make sure they know that the information is available – for example, that all articles published by the team are on the notice board, or that feedback from meetings will be on the locality meeting agenda
- *transparency and probity*: it is important to be absolutely scrupulous about the use of your employer's resources – including your time as well as physical resources. Make sure you have agreed with your manager issues such as whether you are going to a day time meeting in your own time (and if so, need to make up the work time later), or in work time. Similarly establish whether your travel expenses or mileage will be paid by your employer, or if you should claim it back from the organiser of the meeting. Don't use your employer's photocopier, printer or computer for your 'extra' activities such as writing articles or submitting a project for an award, unless you have explicitly checked that you can do so. Don't ask clerical staff to do work on your presentation, or a literature search for your meeting paper, without clarifying that this is acceptable to your (and their) manager. These may seem small things that 'everybody does' – but they are exactly the things that can cause most resentment. More importantly, they are the things that a disgruntled colleague will take note of, and that could lead to embarrassment at best, and disciplinary action at worst, if relationships deteriorate. So get permission, be entirely transparent about what you are doing, and if in doubt, pay for photocopying and phone calls at the time (not later, which suggests a guilty conscience!), or do them elsewhere.

The other factor to be considered at work, apart from colleagues and your manager, is the attitude of the organisation as a whole. Some organisations are very supportive of staff that want to get involved with regional and national initiatives, speak at conferences or write for journals, seeing it as a good reflection on the organisation. However, senior staff are likely to want to keep some control of what is done and said by people in their organisation. You may feel that your organisation is so big that no-one at the top will notice what you are doing – but this is rarely a safe assumption. It is much better to be open and visible in what you are doing: 'they' may not show any interest at all, but at least, if there should be an unexpected problem or reaction, they will not be able to complain that they did not know what you were doing – a position that all senior managers hate to be in.

To avoid problems:

- *work out what attitude your organisation has to external work by looking for precedents*: do other people go to outside forums, sit on national groups, or enter for awards? How is this activity received back at the organisation – is it reported with pride in the in-house magazine, or kept low-key? Are there explicit policies about writing, speaking or undertaking outside activities? Does your manager know what the organisation's attitude is? The more you know, the better you can operate to reduce any problems. If your organisation is completely against these activities, you may need to think about how you balance your ambitions with your future there
- *make sure the right parts of the organisation know what activities you are hoping to engage in*: your manager needs to know, but so may the communications department, a directorate head or senior manager, and the professional development department, if there is one. Apart from the defensive reasons for involving them, it is often very useful to have their help and advice as you embark on influencing activities. They may be able to link you to contacts, or put you in touch with an organisational mentor. And at the very least, you will have raised your profile with some senior people within the organisation, putting yourself on their radar as someone with enthusiasm, dedication and resourcefulness
- *acknowledge permission and help where it is given*: apart from being only polite, this is also much more likely to encourage people to help you, and others, in future
- *report back*: getting permission to go to a regional meeting, or to publish an article, or give a presentation, isn't the end of your obligations to the organisation. You should offer to report back, send a copy of a publication, or summarise responses to your presentation, for the people in your organisation who enabled you to do this
- *establish what should happen to any article or speaking fees your activities generate*: if you did the substantial part of the work in your own time, your organisation may allow you to keep them. Otherwise they may want them to go into a specific fund for staff training, or another specified purpose.

Remember, your success in gaining influence and undertaking outside activities may make your current employer proud and happy to bathe in your reflected glory. Alternatively it may make them anxious that they are going to lose you to a more exciting job, or that you will become 'too hot to handle' because you have such a high profile in your field and you are so busy doing external activities. To maximise the chance of the former, and minimise the latter, it is very important to treat your employing organisation with due respect and consideration.

MIRROR MOMENT

Take time to think through your situation at home and at work. Are the right people aware of your ideas and ambitions? Do you have the time and support you need to undertake at least some of the activities you want to do? If not, would this be a good time to negotiate for change? You will need to ensure that your work, home and extra activities balance out into a reasonable and sustainable way of life.

Consequences from strangers

While a reaction from family, friends and workmates is generally expected when you start to raise your profile in your field of work, the reaction of people you don't know can be quite a surprise. For a start, you – or your name – will be recognised. People will start to send you letters or emails in response to your articles, presentations or input at meetings. You may get requests for site visits, to speak at other events, be interviewed or give advice. Your articles will start to be referenced by other writers, and you may find your words or practice quoted in other people's work. You may secretly love the attention, and think that this is exactly what you wanted to happen – but it can be a mixed blessing.

The good things about this attention are:

- opportunities and contacts start to present themselves to you – you don't have to work so hard to find them
- you have more evidence of the effects of your influencing skills for your portfolio, CV or next job application
- the dialogue with others gives you an incentive to keep up to date, and to develop your knowledge and views
- your profile continues to rise without you doing anything, and the links between you and your subject will get stronger as a result of this cross-referencing.

The downside of this recognition is the nature of some of the reactions you will get from other people. No matter how sound your knowledge, how coherently you express it, and how careful you are of potential pitfalls, you will inevitably offend or annoy somebody, and make mistakes, sooner or later. And they will let you know! It is as well to anticipate both the challenges and demands you will receive from people you don't know, as a consequence of your influencing activities, and learn to respond effectively without taking it too much to heart.

> *Accept that you won't reach or please all of the people all of the time.* (Helen Mould)

Challenges

> *Stick with the difficulties and see them through – be persistent. One of the commonest mistakes is giving up as soon as problems arise.* (Helen McCloughry)

Expect to be challenged on your knowledge, experience and approach to your work. Your personal credibility and your understanding of the subject may be questioned.

Such criticism can become very personal, and feel very wounding. I have had letters from members of my own profession using quite aggressive language: even when they were making a valid point, it could (and should) have been expressed much more professionally.

You may be given a hard time by a questioner at a conference, who seems intent on embarrassing you in front of several hundred people; challenged in a letter to a journal, so that several thousand people see it; or 'put down' with inappropriate comments at a meeting in front of people you have to work with every day. Whatever the reason for such unprofessional behaviour, you have to accept that, if you raise your head above the parapet, it is likely to be shot at, even if there is no obvious reason for doing so.

Sometimes, there will be a reason for the challenge. However good or experienced you are at your work (including influencing work) we all make mistakes or misjudgements sometimes. Raising your profile unfortunately means that more people are likely to notice them!

> *People get really scared of failing. Have five plates spinning, if two crash, you are still ahead of the game.* (HELEN MOULD)

Coping with challenges

> *Admit when you have made a mistake – don't be too concerned about what people think about you personally.* (HELEN MCCLOUGHRY)

First, accept that this will happen. It doesn't mean that you should stop speaking, writing, representing your group or whatever. It doesn't mean that you are wrong – though you may be, and you should always check. But try to grow a thick enough skin that you can deal with challenges without letting them prey on you afterwards.

> *Overall, even the bitchiest person doesn't really want you to fail, and they'll still bitch about you if you succeed . . . so relax.* (ALEXANDRA LEJEUNE)

Then take action. To handle the challenge:

- respond well when it is appropriate to respond (*see* Chapter 19 for meetings, Chapter 21 for presentations, Chapter 22 for conferences and Chapter 23 for letters). No matter how unreasonable or intemperate the challenge, your response should be measured and courteous. Don't escalate situations by hitting back harder, or involving more senior people, however tempting: it only sounds defensive or petulant. Bear in mind that sarcasm really only works in 'real time' and orally. Say it to your computer, but never commit it to paper or email. Take time to review your planned response before sending – 'save as draft' is the most useful instruction on your toolbar at this point!
- acknowledge any genuine mistake you have made – everyone makes mistakes at intervals, and a simple 'yes, you're right' takes the sting out of the challenge
- leave it alone when appropriate (*see* Box 26.1) – sometimes there is no sense in

responding, but this should not be the default option. Some challenges deserve a response, and silence can look like arrogance.

> *A common mistake is giving up at the first setback: you usually have to be persistent and tenacious. If one tactic doesn't work, try another.* (ROSALYNDE LOWE)

BOX 26.1 Examples of challenges that do and do not require a response

It is usually right to respond to:

- *an accusation of a technical mistake or wrong information*: if it is wrong it needs to be corrected; if not, you need to clear up the confusion for the person, and the rest of the readership/audience
- *a misinterpretation of your organisation or group's position*: you need to defend the group's reputation
- *a request for information, however ungraciously couched*: otherwise you risk further inflaming the grievance.

It is usually better *not* to respond to:

- *a statement of a contrary opinion to your own*: the challenger is entitled to their own opinion, and unless you really want a dialogue, it is difficult to close it down if you start to exchange opinions
- *a dismissive or insulting comment*: unless actually libellous and damaging; even then, you may simply prolong and enlarge its exposure
- *repeated challenges*: if someone is determined to have the last word, it is quicker and less stressful to let them.

Demands

The other consequence of visibility in your field is the demands that people make on you. Health and social care is a remarkably small world, in spite of its vast workforce; and somehow there are never enough people willing to represent a group, lead change, write or speak. Look at national conference programmes for any clinical or service area, and you will see the same names coming up repeatedly. So raising your profile is likely to lead to lots of invitations to take on more work or extra activities. To manage this:

- keep reviewing the match between your 'day job' and your other activities: there may come a time when you need to change one or other
- check back with your manager or team if outside demands mean that you are going to be away from your workplace more often: permission or tolerance for your initial extra commitments will not automatically extend to accommodate the growth in demand
- consider putting explicit limits on the demands you will respond to: accepting speaking engagements no more than once a quarter; agreeing to sit on a group for a year only; chairing a forum on a rotating basis with another member. This

may be useful for your own sake, but is also helpful to reassure your manager or your team that you recognise your responsibility to them and are actively ensuring that you can deliver on it.

Practical consequences of exposure

There are a few practical things that you need to pay attention to when you are undertaking 'outside' work:

- *income tax*: remember if you are keeping fees for writing or speaking, that you need to declare the extra income for tax purposes – however small it might seem. Keep a record of expenses associated with the activity, which can be offset against the income
- *claiming fees and expenses*: keep receipts for expenses that you will claim from third parties (not your employer) separate from your other expenses, so that you can demonstrate clearly that you are claiming appropriately. Photocopy any expense forms and receipts you send to other organisations – they have a habit of getting lost, and it is even more difficult to deal with the finance departments of organisations you don't work for, than to get expenses out of your employer. Create your own invoice template for claiming fees from bodies that don't have standard expense claim forms, and save copies of each one sent out. Check regularly that you have received what you have claimed for – invoices can move very slowly through systems and it is easy to forget them as the months pass
- *record keeping*: if your professional portfolio is bulging, keep a separate file for published articles, the reports on your award-winning project, or papers for the forum you lead. But cross reference to your portfolio so that you will remember to put all the relevant activities on a job application or CV.

PORTFOLIO POINTER

Keep conference programmes as an easy reminder of what you spoke about, when, where and to whom – it is quicker than writing a list.

CHECKLIST FOR ACTION

Have you:

- talked to your manager and relevant colleagues about any external activities you are undertaking/want to undertake?
- established how you will handle 'time owing' and miscellaneous expenses?
- put expenses and record-keeping systems in place, as computer or hard-copy files?

CHAPTER 27

Endings

Never burn your boats, you never know when or where someone might re-appear. (Deb Lapthorne)

Imagine that you have achieved your ambitions regarding influence. You have a profile in your area of work or practice; you are regularly asked to attend meetings, join groups, lead projects, write articles and speak at conferences. You are on first-name terms with leaders in practice and policy, who periodically exchange information and views with you. What happens next?

Going 'inside'

You may continue to develop these activities, running your 'public' life alongside your day job, making adjustments and compromises where necessary. Or you may choose to move into a job where they are the stuff of your day-to-day work, rather than 'add ons'. Posts in clinical leadership or management, or in strategy or policy organisations, provide these opportunities. It is as well to be aware, though, that working in such a post will feel entirely different to contributing from 'outside'. Instead of being the talented and respected expert, brought in to advise or share with others, you become just another insider, with all the institutional and cultural issues to deal with. Some people make the transition very successfully, but others find that full-time work of this kind is not for them, and revert to doing their influencing from a practice or service base. If you have chance to test out the difference before making the change permanently– by taking on a secondment, or doing a job swap – this is a very good idea.

Taking a break

There is also likely to come a time when you want or need to reduce or even stop some of your influencing activities. Common reasons are:

- a change in your job, reducing time or opportunity
- a change in your family circumstances
- illness or another crisis requiring your full attention for a lengthy period.

> *One of the most important factors in developing my career was being true to myself and being very clear about the point beyond which I was not prepared to compromise.* (Deb Lapthorne)

Giving up activities for any of these (or other) reasons does not constitute a failure, or even a backward step: you are simply recognising the need to rebalance your activities. Having a positive exit strategy helps to demonstrate this to yourself and to others.

In addition to these practical reasons, there are more internal reasons for deciding to call a halt to some influencing activities. You may find that you are bored with 'your' subject, or becoming complacent and stale in speaking about it. You may feel that you are becoming 'type-cast' – so closely associated with a particular subject area that you are under-rated (and perhaps under-informed and lacking confidence) in others. Even if you are still enjoying the activities of influencing, it may be time to change subject or focus in order to continue to be involved, and to continue building your reputation. Bear in mind also that your credibility may wane over time, particularly if you spend more and more time away from direct involvement with clients or patients. So a change of direction, a period of refreshing skills and paying attention to the service delivery workplace can be positively helpful to your future influence.

Managing your exit

The key to leaving, whether a job, editorial board, advisory group or project team, is to do it so well that everyone is immediately desperate to have you back! This sounds obvious, but is done surprisingly rarely. It is odd that people who are so keen to get into committees, speak to ministers or publish in journals can be so casual about ending their involvement. Some common examples of bad practice that I have come across are:

- failing to attend meetings for months without ever sending any explanation
- getting their PA to email to say that they are too busy to continue contributing to a reference group
- announcing that they are leaving a post, and so no longer available to continue contributing to a piece of work, with only a couple of weeks' notice and at a critical point
- leaving the executive committee of a forum and taking all the shared papers and books with them
- assuming they will never see these people again and becoming rude and careless
- implying that they have 'grown out of' the work and have something better to do.

MIRROR MOMENT

Think about times that you have left a job or stopped contributing to a piece of work or a group. Did you manage to end it well, or did you do any of the above?

Most of us have been guilty of one or other of these at some time, particularly the passive ones like failing to attend meetings. What would you do differently next time, in order to have a positive influence on your reputation and legacy?

Good endings

Naturally, the way to ensure that people continue to think well of you and want to involve you in future is to do the opposite of the above! It is always worth the effort. Not only does it stop that nagging guilt when you know you should have acted differently, it also keeps the way open for future opportunities. This is very important in health and social care: in spite of the huge workforce, it is an astonishingly small world. You *will* meet those people again, or at least go for a job, to a meeting or to a conference with someone who knows one of them. Reputations travel, and people make judgements on what they hear. This is how you were invited into your various influencing activities in the first place, so it shouldn't be surprising if it also works the other way. Unreliability, discourtesy and lack of consideration at the end of a piece of work will undo all the credibility gained when you were new to it, keen and responsive.

So, a few important things to do to make a good exit:

- *give as much warning as possible*, to allow for the identification and recruitment of a replacement on the group, board or project, or a new speaker/presenter for the meeting or conference. The politest email in the world will not offset the effect of pulling out at 24 hours' notice
- *give a reason for ending your involvement*. Honesty is good: if you need to give more time to your job, or you feel you are becoming stale and someone else could contribute more, it is as well to say so. Lying is not good, and may be found out. Saying that your organisation is stopping you, you have a new, more demanding job or you are emigrating to Australia, is a dangerous tactic if it is not true. But if the reason is personal and sensitive, you can adopt a cliché ('personal reasons', 'ill-health') and stick to it. Giving no reason at all feels like a rebuff to the person or organisation you are withdrawing from, and leaves an ambiguous feeling about you at best. So do explain, even if in minimal terms
- *tell the right person first*: the chair of a meeting, board or committee, even if your most frequent contact is with the secretary. Then make sure that all the relevant people who need to know are told, including the secretary
- *offer to help find a successor*: this may not be accepted, but shows that you care enough about the work you were involved in to try. If the offer is accepted, do your best to find someone suitable. Be objective about this: remember your successor, like someone who deputises for you, reflects on you and your organisation. It is not a time to gift the place to a friend, or name just anyone so that you can say you helped. The new person needs to fit the bill for the work, otherwise both your and their reputation will suffer

You need to bring people along with you so that if you leave then the change does not leave with you. (Judith Whittam)

- *offer to hand back any unique information or resources you were given as part of your role in this work*: other than meeting notes and similar, which everyone in the group received. If you are disposing of information, make sure you treat confidential material appropriately, shredding papers and deleting emails
- *write a final letter or email to the chair*, or your most senior contact, to confirm that you are ending your involvement. Give the reason, thank them for the opportunity, and mention how it has helped you (learned new skills, understand field better, met very helpful people) and how you will use this (better able to develop your service, will benefit your patients, clients or students). Add the practical details – date of finishing, what you have done about returning materials, etc. This is good manners and enhances your reputation – but is also a useful insurance for you. If questions are asked in future, about who had access to leaked information or whether you returned a piece of equipment, or if you want to dissociate yourself from actions or decisions taken after you had left – then your leaving letter is a very useful piece of evidence.

PERSONAL DEVELOPMENT EXERCISE

Jot down an exit plan for a piece of influencing work you are currently engaged in. Make a checklist of who you will write to, what resources you would return, what information you will need to dispose of, and which contacts you will want to keep. Then file it in your professional portfolio until the time comes to end your involvement in that piece of work.

Reaping the rewards of a good exit

It almost takes less time to do these things than it does to describe them, and will reap benefits in the future. When I joined the Department of Health in 1999, I had to withdraw from membership of three editorial advisory boards, the writing of two regular columns in nursing journals, membership of the professional executive committee of a professional association, and talks with the publisher about writing this book, as well as my day job. It required a lot of letters and explanations, and seemed to take a lot of time and effort at the time. But six years later, when I was ready to pick up on these kinds of activities, I believe my warm reception on all of these fronts was because I had taken trouble to exit professionally when I had to. People do remember!

PORTFOLIO POINTER

Put copies of your 'exit' letter or email into your portfolio, to remind you of the things you have been involved in, and the dates you finished. The wording is also useful years later when you want to put something in a job application about what you learned from your activities. If you receive letters of thanks from your contacts in response to your leaving (as you should), file these too. They are heartening to read in future just to make yourself feel better when times are tough, but they also provide good quotes for future CVs.

Keeping the contacts

Finally, before you close the book on that particular activity, make sure you have recorded contact details of key people you met in the course of the work. They can remain part of your network even if you are not working directly with them, and, in the small world of healthcare, it is very likely that you will want to talk to them, or they to you, in the future.

CHECKLIST FOR ACTION

Have you:

- produced an exit plan for future use for an activity you are involved in?

Summary

If you have read this book by dipping into chapters that seem relevant, the summary list below will remind you of other areas you might want to look at – or it may reassure you that you have all the skills and information you need to be astutely aware and effectively influential.

The top ten tips for awareness and influence

Awareness

1. Get good at email, word processing and web searching.
2. Build a wide network and keep adding to it.
3. Read more journals, newspapers and policy documents.
4. Get at least one mentor and work actively with them.
5. Become an expert in a specific topic.

Influence

1. Use meetings for networking as well as business.
2. Write articles in a range of journals.
3. Put in abstracts for papers, workshops and posters at conferences.
4. Write to key people in your field.
5. Join or start a group or network.

I hope the ideas, tips and information in this book, and the insights from the many expert contributors, have helped you realise your ambitions to influence your part of health and social care. Services, patients and communities should be the better for it.

INDEX